A Trip to Labrador

A Trip to Labrador

Letters and Journal
of
Edward Caldwell Moore

EDITED & INTRODUCED BY
KIRBY WALSH

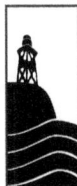

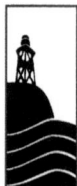

BREAKWATER BOOKS LTD.
JESPERSON PUBLISHING • BREAKWATER DISTRIBUTORS
w w w . b r e a k w a t e r b o o k s . c o m

Library and Archives Canada Cataloguing in Publication

Walsh, Kirby, 1941-

Moore, Edward Caldwell, 1857-1943
   A trip to Labrador : letters and journals of Edward Caldwell Moore /
   edited & introduced by Kirby Walsh.

Includes bibliographical references and index.
ISBN 978-1-55081-252-7

1. Moore, Edward Caldwell, 1857-1943--Correspondence.
2. Moore, Edward Caldwell, 1857-1943--Diaries.
3. Labrador (N.L.)--Description and travel.
4. Grenfell, Wilfred Thomason, Sir, 1865-1940. 5. Missions, Medical--Newfoundland
and Labrador--Labrador--History.
I. Walsh, Kirby II. Title.

FC2193.51.M66 2009   971.8'202092   C2009-900833-5

Edward Caldwell Moore's letters and journal, as well as the front and back cover photos of Edward
Caldwell Moore, are used with permission from the Andover-Harvard Theological Library,
Harvard Divinity School, Cambridge, Massachusetts, and from Sandy Moore Bureau.

Photos in insert are used with permission from *Them Days: Stories of Early Labrador* Inc., Labrador
Archives, Happy Valley-Goose Bay, and the Andover-Harvard Theological Library, Harvard
Divinity School, Cambridge, Massachusetts.

The Canada Council | Le Conseil des Arts
  for the Arts | du Canada

We acknowledge the financial support of The Canada Council for the Arts for
our publishing activities.

We acknowledge the support of the Department of Tourism, Culture and
Recreation for our publishing activities.

Newfoundland
Labrador

We acknowledge the financial support of the Government of Canada through
the Book Publishing Industry Development Program (BPIDP) for our publishing activities.

Canada

Printed in Canada

CONTENTS

INTRODUCTION

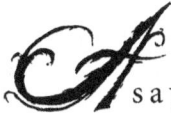

As a young man of twenty-seven, Edward Caldwell Moore, a Presbyterian minister and, subsequently, a Harvard professor, studied in Germany for two years at the post-graduate level. There, he no doubt learned about and possibly talked with the Moravians (founded in Saxony by emigrants from Moravia and with headquarters in eastern Germany) who had initiated the first large-scale Protestant missionary movement. Their care for the poor inspired the sending of missionaries, both clergy and laity, to various corners of the world, including northern Labrador. Moore was impressed with their work in missionary outreach, and his curiosity about Moravian missions may have prompted him to take the opportunity to visit Labrador in 1905 and see, first-hand, Moravian settlements and missionary work with native peoples. His interest in the work of Wilfred Grenfell also may have been a factor.

Dr. Wilfred Grenfell had visited Boston and New York in 1897 on one of his North American lecture tours to make people more aware of the needs of the scattered population on the Labrador coast and to raise money to improve social and medical conditions there. In the winter of 1905, he was in the Boston area again, for the same purpose, and he visited the home of Edward Caldwell Moore and his family. At that time, Grenfell extended an invitation for Moore to visit with him on the Labrador coast in the summer, to travel by boat among the fishing stations, and to see the conditions that existed among the fishermen and their families. Moore determined that he would undertake such a journey, not merely as a visitor or as a tourist, but as a pilgrim, to take part in the work of the mission, to participate in and lead worship, and to help Grenfell in any ways that presented during the cruise.

This offer to Moore was by no means unique, for Grenfell was well known for issuing such invitations. During this same lecture tour, he invited a Jessie Luther to come north and set up a handicrafts enterprise, which she did the following year. Another example: The Rev. Henry Gordon, at that time a well-known Church of England minister serving the Cartwright area, spoke of Grenfell in his journal, *The Labrador Parson*, saying: "It was, in fact, at his invitation that I went out to Labrador" (p.1). In the ten years that he served that region, whenever possible, Gordon met with Grenfell and they spent time together during Grenfell's summer trips along the Labrador coast.

Moore, in 1905, was Parkman Professor of Theology at Harvard, and Grenfell had a long association with that university. In his autobiography, *A Labrador Doctor*, Grenfell mentioned: "A member of my own profession, the Professor of Physiology of Harvard University, by name Alexander Forbes, a lifelong friend…" (p. 255). No doubt, such friends had a great deal of influence regarding the needs of the mission and made it easier for Grenfell to recruit help from physicians for summer work along the Labrador coast. Moore mentions a Dr. Crockett, aurist, of Boston, who had served with Grenfell. Dr. Rufus A. Kingman was there at the same time as Moore, and Dr. Alexander McKenzie was also mentioned as being present. Then, of course, there were numerous others who answered Grenfell's invitation to visit and to serve on the Labrador. Moore's trip, however, was different from the others in that he would write extensively about his experiences and these writings would be preserved in letters and a journal.

There was at least one other person, however, who wrote of his experiences with Grenfell and sent a journal to his family: Eliot Curwen. Grenfell had invited the young medical missionary to help him on the Labrador during 1893, his second year on the coast. Curwen kept a journal from May 27 to November 18 of that year, which he sent home to England in instalments. This journal was edited by Ronald Rompkey and published as *Labrador Odyssey*, with additional material, in 1996.

Moore was keenly interested in Grenfell's stories and descriptions of life on the Labrador. Further interest was created by Grenfell's and others' writings of people, places and events, and plans for serving the people of Labrador. Magazines such as *Among the Deep Sea Fishers* and books such as *Doctor Luke of the Labrador* were known to Moore and increased his interest in this area. During his journey, he also read *The Lure of the Labrador Wild* by Dillon Wallace, the story of the ill-fated Leonidas Hubbard expedition.

In the spring, Moore talked with Dr. Crockett, who had experienced Labrador previously with Grenfell, about what to expect, and he made plans to go north in the summer of 1905. Moore followed Crockett's advice about what he would see and what he should take on such a journey. He wrote of his preparations in his letters from Cambridge to his wife at Orange, a small town north of Boston, expressing his satisfaction with how things were progressing and how much money he would have to spend. He showed some concern in leaving his family for this extended period and anticipated some loneliness on both sides. He was actually away from his family from July 13 to September 4, when he arrived back in Boston and went to meet them the next day.

In mid-July, Moore travelled on the ferry S.S. *Olivette* to Halifax, Nova Scotia, and on to Port Hawkesbury, Cape Breton. From there he went by train to Sydney, Cape Breton, and joined the S.S. *Bruce*, the ferry to Port aux Basques, Newfoundland. A narrow-gauge railway then took him to Bay of Islands to connect with the ferry to Battle Harbour, Labrador. At that time the coastal steamer S.S. *Home* was the ferry serving that area from Humbermouth, now Corner Brook. At Battle Harbour, Moore met with Dr. Grenfell and visited the hospital there. Next, they journeyed south to St. Anthony and the surrounding area and then north along the Labrador coast to the hospital at Indian Harbour and as far as Black Island, twenty-five miles northeast of Nain. At Nain and at Makkovik and Hopedale, he was successful in visiting the Moravian Mission and native settlements, one of the chief interests of his trip.

Moore described his experiences in his letters, almost daily, to his wife, and after travelling beyond the regular mail area for the post office, he continued to write a daily journal. He described the difficulty in making mail and ferry connections in those days and his frustrations at not having a definite schedule for mail as for everything else. He wrote of the stark conditions experienced by those who lived on the Labrador year-round and by those who ventured there in schooners during the summer cod-fishing season. He learned of the deprivation of the people through lack of medical services and of the misery which often occurred when the fishery failed. He talked personally with people who worked on the Labrador and with others who came for Dr. Grenfell's medical attention. Moore was a man of his times. He spoke with prejudice about a Jewish peddler, and when he met the native people of Labrador, the Inuit and Innu, who needed medical attention or were starving, he wrote of their plight with great empathy, but he also occasionally used terms we would now consider disparaging and offensive.

It seems that Moore was unprepared for the extent of the isolation he experienced in northern Labrador. At times, he may have been fearful for his own safety in the wilds surrounded by ice and fog. His sense of separation from his family was acute at these times, as his letters and journals testify. In Labrador in 1905, as still today, one had to wait upon the weather being favourable, the tides being right, and the Arctic ice conditions being suitable for travel. Sometimes this resulted in extended periods of waiting and frustration as schedules went out the window and one and all could but curse the elements or pray for better weather.

His personal experience of Dr. Grenfell's work and administrative decisions left Moore questioning Grenfell's competency in some areas. While he admired Grenfell's hard work and commitment in his chosen field of medicine, he could have appreciated more the difficult and demanding conditions under which decisions had to be made in a land devoid of schedules and security. However, his descriptions of Grenfell's humanity and foibles are quite refreshing, and one gets the impression that he is writing about a real person who is never one-dimensional. The reader sees another side of Grenfell, in addition to that of the medical hero of early Labrador.

Here, we see two persons of very different character. Moore is a Presbyterian minister as well as a Harvard professor. His Protestant theology did not always agree with Grenfell's Church of England, evangelical grounding. Moore was aware that it is much easier to observe liturgical decorum in a chapel at Harvard than on board a ship off the coast of Labrador. Grenfell, partly because he had more experience through his work on the Labrador and in the North Sea, was more likely than Moore to be impressed with the impromptu services of worship and hymn-singing on Sunday evenings observed on the decks of many fishing schooners at anchor in the harbours along the Labrador coast. It was reported that the captains would lead the worship and the lusty notes of the crews could easily be heard from shore as they sang together the very meaningful—for them at the time—words of the hymn, "Will your anchor hold in the storms of life?"

Grenfell, in his autobiography *A Labrador Doctor*, describes a sealing voyage he undertook to the "Front," an area off the northeast coast of Newfoundland, on board the S.S. *Neptune* in March 1896. He reported that on Sunday afternoon the whole crew assembled on deck, sang hymns, and "had Evening Prayer together, Catholic and Protestant alike; and for my part I felt the nearness of God's presence as really as I have felt it in the mysterious environment of the most magnificent cathedral" (p.124).[1] Grenfell always included other religious denominations in his approach to spirituality. His was an ecumenical attitude. He worked with others regardless of their religious orientation.

Moore was impressed with the fact that, although the fishing season was so short (from June to October), very few of the crews worked on Sundays. He was unaware that there could be a practical reason for this as well as a religious one. A crew with a weekly day of rest will, over the course of the summer, produce more fish than a crew working seven days a week all through the season. The six-day week maintains a noticeably higher psychical and physical energy level among the crew, and the production will be greater. I noticed this during several seasons of fishing on the Labrador coast in the 1950s. One Friday evening, for example, our crew had a boatload of fish at the stage head and more in the cod-bag. We decided to work all night. By noon on Saturday we found that our production rate had dropped noticeably. By suppertime it was decided to knock off early. We did not repeat that experience, recognizing that human energy can be spread only so far.

---

[1] For another description of this service see George Whiteley's *Northern Seas, Hardy Sailors*, p. 51.

Moore's observations offer a fresh perspective, for he experienced Grenfell and his mission in the early days when Grenfell was still creating the legend of the Labrador doctor. As one who was born at Cartwright and grew up on the Labrador, I have heard several of the older generation speak of Dr. Grenfell and express appreciation for his work. Always, the work that was mentioned was his pioneering efforts in setting up hospitals at strategic centres and travelling the coast to doctor those in need who lived far from these centres.

When Moore visited Turnavik on the north Labrador coast he found the fishermen there experiencing a difficult season because of drift ice. The cod fish had come in but the traps could not be set. They had no fish. This was always a problem on the Labrador. Fishermen experienced similar summers at Pack's Harbour on the south Labrador coast. One year in particular in the early 1960s, the ice forced us to take up the cod traps in early July. Instead of sitting around and waiting, we got out the jiggers (usually reserved until after the trapping season). For the next few days we jigged, from around the ice pans, an average of twenty to thirty quintals per day—little more than enough to pay expenses—but far short of the eighty to one hundred and ten quintals we averaged from the trap on a good day.

In the 1950s and early '60s, when I fished for cod at Indian Tickle with my uncle, Jim Burdett, and later for cod and then salmon at Pack's Harbour, outside Cartwright, with my father, Billy Walsh, conditions on the Labrador were no different from half a century earlier. The work was just as hard, the hours just as long, and the returns barely adequate. The credit system, in which the merchant supplied the fishing gear, food, and salt, was still in effect, and at the end of the season, with salt-bulk fish at only five dollars a quintal (112 lbs.), even the "high-liner" fishermen barely made a living.

Grenfell was concerned about the credit system because he felt that merchants were in a position to take advantage of the fishermen. That they sometimes did was attested to by an incident related by my father who described how, one fall, he went into the office of Baine, Johnson and Company in Battle Harbour (owner of the fishing premises in Battle Harbour from 1871 to the early 1950s) to "straighten up" after a summer of fishing in Indian Cove. He was informed by the merchant that one of the items he had "charged" was a carton of cigarettes. He immediately denied this, saying: "I have never charged cigarettes in my life." After looking intensely at him for a minute the merchant replied: "Well, if you didn't, somebody else did," and he wrote the cigarettes, arbitrarily, on another's account.

Some social and economic conditions, however, *had* changed, and in the 1950s and '60s, for example, nearly everyone owned a "make-and-break" engine, and the labour-intensive work of rowing the big, heavy trap-boats was a thing of the past. Transportation was easier but people in the small fishing communities still had far to travel for medical attention. Many relied on the coastal boats, notably the S.S. *Kyle*, to get them to doctors at St. Anthony, Mary's Harbour, Cartwright, North West River, or Happy Valley-Goose Bay. In critical emergencies, an aircraft might be used when the weather was favourable, and emergency medical evacuations were carried out by bush-pilots flying in from the larger centres. Regular visits were made along the coast by doctors in Grenfell hospital ships, such as Dr. William Anthony Paddon's trips during his many years on the *Maravel*. So, on the whole, this area of people's lives saw gradual improvement.

It is not surprising that such a sparse population in such a big land would see little change in other areas over half a century. The collapse of the northern cod-fishery in the 1970s, however, and the construction of the Trans-Labrador Highway (nearing completion in 2008) are different stories for they have brought many ongoing changes to the lives of the people of the Labrador coast.

Moore made a few dire predictions about Grenfell's work, and he was not alone in such predictions. For example, Tim Borlase in *The Labrador Settlers, Métis and Kablunângajuit* gives a picture of how Grenfell was perceived by some in his own time. As part of his descriptions of the "Founding of the Grenfell Mission," Borlase writes: "The promises and activities of the Grenfell Association made many friends but it made many enemies too. Because Wilfred Grenfell often attacked the status quo (that is, the way things were), he drew the anger of many authorities and institutions of the day. Merchants, liquor traders and even some church leaders exploited the very people they claimed to serve. These authorities felt threatened by Grenfell's accomplishments, and spent much time finding fault with them" (p. 207). Consequently, several merchants made a petition to the government demanding an investigation, and this petition resulted in the Squarey Commission of 1917. Robert T. Squarey, District Magistrate for the St. Anthony District, which included Labrador, chaired a Royal Commission to inquire into allegations made against charities operating on the Labrador coast, namely, the Grenfell Mission. Although there was no legal business connection between the Co-operative Stores and the International Grenfell Association, Grenfell is listed in a "Directory of Company Directors," as Director of the "Spot Cash Co-operative Co., Ltd."[2] This made him answerable to the Commission for any allegations against the Co-operatives as well as against the IGA. The merchants had alleged that the IGA portrayed Newfoundlanders as paupers, that charities were in unfair competition with merchants, that Co-operative Stores were subsidized by Americans, and that charities had committed breaches of the Customs Act. However, in his final report of November 1, 1917, as chair of the Commission, Magistrate Squarey praised the work of the IGA and completely exonerated Grenfell from any wrong doing. Possibly, Moore, in his observations of Grenfell, anticipated such troubles.

In his letter to his son, Moore speaks of the viciousness of some of the Labrador huskies. I've had first-hand experience of the truth of that observation. At the age of about four or five I was playing on the slippery ice below a high bank in Mary's Harbour with my cousin, Denley Cumby. I was lying on the ice and Denley was standing just a few feet away. Suddenly, I saw a husky dog skid along by my feet. It was a big, white one that had trouble stopping on the slippery ice. I tried to jump up but another dog grabbed my face and another my legs, and I was immediately covered by a whole team of seven or eight dogs. Lucky for me the dogs' owner saw them running and came to my rescue. I spent several days in the hospital and still have the scars to show. The owner killed all the dogs, a great loss to him, because he, too, could not trust them now. Denley escaped unharmed although he would have made a better meal, skinny

---

[2] Joseph R. Smallwood, ed., *The Book of Newfoundland*. Vol. 2, p. 319.

as I was. Perhaps the dogs thought I was a seal lying on the ice, a costly mistake for me and for them.

Moore wrote of the difficulty of getting stove-wood to Battle Harbour Island from the mainland. Keeping the houses heated, especially in winter, involved much work and much time in transportation. There were dangers, too. When we lived in Indian Cove, a few miles across Caribou Island from Battle Harbour, I heard my father relate an incident in which, one fall he and his father went up St. Lewis Bay for a boatload of wood. They overloaded the boat that calm day with the intention of unloading some of the wood at the mouth of the bay and thereby saving several miles on the next trip. However, when they came to the mouth of the bay they decided to continue on to Indian Cove with the full load. A strong breeze of northeast wind sprung up and they narrowly escaped being swamped. Years later, as a small boy, I went with my father by dog-team from Indian Cove across the tickle to the mainland for a komatik load of wood. The salt-water ice had only a couple of nights' frost, and on the way back the loaded komatik pushed a very noticeable wave of buckling ice ahead of her nose. I remember my father warning me to stay on the komatik and urging the team on. We got safely across, thanks to the flexibility of the salt-water ice—some refer to it as "rubber ice"—which buckled but did not break.

It is interesting to note that Grenfell was aware of Moore's writing and must have read at least some of it. In *A Labrador Doctor*, he quotes from Moore's letter of July 26 and journal of August 21 in a reference to the foxes that he (Grenfell) had procured for his fox-farm at St. Anthony. He writes: "A Harvard Professor who happened to be cruising with me that summer records that I was carrying fifteen little foxes…" (p. 158). Grenfell continues further to quote Moore's descriptions of the foxes. Whether or not Grenfell read all of the journal, he did not say, but it seems likely that he did. I am unaware of whether or not that reading affected their relationship in any way.

As revising editor, in typing the manuscript of Moore's letters and journal, I have preserved as true a rendition of his script as possible. I have kept his punctuation, capitals, abbreviations, and sequence, but have corrected obvious misspellings. I have guessed at a few words that were impossible for me to decipher; these I have enclosed in brackets. The use of an ellipsis indicates that I have been unable to read two or more words in one sentence. I have not included the year—1905—in the heading of each letter as Moore did. For clarity, I have added italics to ships' names, and I have footnoted where an observation might provide additional information. All references, page numbers, and so forth noted in footnotes refer to materials listed in the bibliography. Everything within brackets in the following letters and journal, as well as the footnotes, biographical notes, index, headings and summaries, are the words and work of the revising editor. Any errors or omissions in the following text are also mine alone.

Moore was writing extensively—in indelible pencil—and composing his thoughts, without revision, as he proceeded to put them to paper. He often summarized sentences, for example, "Was much interested in…" He used a form of shorthand, such as wh for which, wd for would, shd for should, G. for Grenfell, and so forth. For the most part, Moore used American spellings for harbour (harbor), colour (color), odour (odor), and so forth. I have retained these spellings. The reader, therefore, can expect a different text than might be written in modern Canadian English.

Moore was, no doubt, sometimes influenced in his writing by rough conditions at sea and sometimes by the stress of the journey and the pressure to be concise. He recorded much information in a very short time. Sometimes, he ended his letters abruptly because he had run out of space on the page, or he continued to write around the margins. In his letters from China, which came more than a year later, he wrote vertically over some pages where he had already written horizontally: a wonderful way to save paper, no doubt, but it may try the patience of the reader!

The letters all have very formal salutations and signatures, such as "My Dear Wife," and, "Your Husband, Edward C. Moore." Even his letter to his son is signed, "Your Father, Edward C. Moore." Moore's final Labrador letter to his wife is dated August 8 from Indian Harbour. This was his last opportunity to send mail to her that would arrive before he returned; after this, his writing is in journal form.

Some of the comments in the letters to his wife are of a personal nature and irrelevant to the Labrador trip itself; these I have omitted. For example, on Friday, July 28, he wrote from the *Strathcona*: "My Dearest Wife: We will not count this letter as one of the series." There followed a personal letter with a few references to his journey but much is irrelevant to the context. His comment here seems to imply that he may have been considering producing his letters and journal for a wider audience.

Despite the disappointing ending of his trip, Edward Caldwell Moore's brief time in Labrador in 1905 produced the following observations and comments, some factual and some "hear-say," that have brought forward another slice of history for those interested in early life on the Labrador.

His letters and journal, as well as other papers and photographs, were donated to the Andover-Harvard Theological Library in 1971 by his daughter, Dr. Dorothea May Moore (Mrs. Arthur Burkhardt).

EDWARD CALDWELL MOORE:
BIOGRAPHICAL NOTES

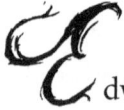

dward Caldwell Moore was born in West Chester, Pennsylvania, in 1857, the son of William E. Moore and Harriet Foot Moore.

Moore completed his liberal arts education at Marietta College, Marietta, Ohio, receiving an A.B. (from the Latin, *Artium Baccalaureus*) and an A.M. (*Artium Magister*) in 1880. He decided to study for ministry in the Presbyterian Church and entered Union Theological Seminary in New York, which was founded in 1836 under the auspices of the Presbyterian Church. He received a B.D. (Bachelor of Divinity) from Union in 1884 and was ordained a Presbyterian minister in that same year.

On November 9, 1887, Moore married Eliza Coe Brown, daughter of John Crosby Brown of New York and Mary Elizabeth (Adams) Brown. He sometimes addressed his wife in his correspondence, affectionately, as "Bessie."

Three children were born to them. First, a daughter, whom they named Dorothea May, was born May 13, 1894. Her father sometimes referred to her in his correspondence as "Dorry." Dr. Dorothea May Moore (Mrs. Arthur Burkhardt) lived to be more than one hundred years of age and died in 1995. Her niece, Sandys Moore Bureau, remembers that she maintained a life-long interest in the work of the Grenfell Mission. A son, John Crosby Brown Moore, was born April 12, 1897. John grew up to become an architect. He died in June 1993, at the age of ninety-six, leaving one child, Sandys Moore Bureau. His obituary stated that he was well known in New York as a designer of university buildings, churches, and civic institutions. In his letter from Labrador, his father addressed him as "Hans." Their last child was a daughter, Elizabeth Ripley Moore. She was born January 29, 1907, and died leaving one child, Stark Ward.

Moore was academically inclined and became involved in extensive post-graduate education. He studied in Germany at the universities of Berlin, Gottingen, and Giessen from 1884 to 1886. Then, from 1886 to 1889, he served as Presbyterian minister in Yonkers, New York, the fourth largest city in the state of New York, located two miles north of Manhattan. Afterwards, he held a two-year pastorate, 1889 to 1901, at Central Congregational Church, Providence, Rhode Island.

Moore was granted a Ph.D. from Brown University in Providence, Rhode Island, in 1891. In 1892, he was awarded an Honorary D.D. from Marietta College and, in 1909, an Honorary D.D. from Yale University in New Haven, Connecticut. In 1920, he earned an LL.D. from Grinnell College in Grinnell, Iowa, a college with a strong tradition of social activism. He completed a D.Th. from the University of Giessen in Germany in 1926.

In 1901, Moore began teaching at Harvard University, the oldest institution of higher learning in the United States. In that capacity, as Parkman Professor of Theology, he preached at Appleton Chapel, Harvard, for twenty-two years.

At the invitation of Sir Wilfred Grenfell in 1905, Moore journeyed to Newfoundland and Labrador, and in 1907, February to April, he undertook a trip to China on behalf of the Prudential Committee of The American Board of Commissioners for Foreign Missions. As he had on the earlier trip to Labrador, Moore again wrote extensively to his wife, and these letters also have been preserved at Andover-Harvard Theological Library.

He became Chairman of the Board of Preachers and Plummer Professor of Christian Morals at Harvard in 1915. From 1914 to 1925 he was President of the American Board of Commissioners for Foreign Missions. During this time he was an occasional visiting lecturer at various colleges: Andover Seminary, Yale Divinity School, The Lowell Institute, and Mansfield College, Oxford.

Moore specialized in the Reformation and Post-Reformation

periods, as well as in the philosophy of religion. He authored several books and papers including: *The New Testament in the Christian Church*, 1904; "The Naturalization of Christianity in the Far East," *The Harvard Theological Review*. Vol. 1 (3), 1908; *An Outline of the History of Christian Thought since Kant*, 1913; *West and East; The Nature of Religion; The Spread of Christianity in the Modern World*, 1919; "The Christian Doctrine of Nature," *The Journal of Religion*. Vol. 3 (1), 1923; "A Century of Unitarianism in the United States," *The Journal of Religion*. Vol. 5 (4), 1925.

Moore's papers include a long list of addresses, college lectures, and articles: there are prayers, sermons, and correspondences, including family and general letters and photographs. These were all donated to Andover-Harvard Theological Library in 1971 by his daughter Dorothea [Edward Caldwell Moore, Letters from Labrador, bMS 422/7 and bMS 638/6, Andover-Harvard Theological Library, Harvard Divinity School, Cambridge, Massachusetts].

Edward Caldwell Moore, A.B., A.M., B.D., Ph.D., D.D., LL.D., D.Th., died in 1943 at the age of eighty-six.

SIR WILFRED THOMASON GRENFELL:
BIOGRAPHICAL NOTES

In researching the following information some discrepancies were found in dates and spelling. Whenever that was the case, I followed the information in Grenfell's own autobiography.

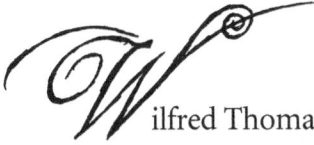

ilfred Thomason Grenfell was born February 28, 1865, at Parkgate, England. He was the son of The Rev. Algernon Sydney Grenfell and his wife Jane.

Grenfell attended Oxford University for a brief time, then he enrolled at London Hospital Medical College in February 1883. He joined the Royal National Mission to Deep Sea Fishermen, established in the early 1880s as a British, evangelical, medical mission to fishermen in the North Sea. The organization also provided financial, emotional and pastoral support to fishermen's families in the United Kingdom and Isle of Man.

Grenfell's first visit to the Labrador coast was made in the medical ship *Albert* in 1892. This visit was followed by a lecture tour of England to raise funds for medical work on the coast. In 1893, he established a seasonal hospital at Battle Harbour, which, the following year, remained open all year. He did a lecture tour of Canada. Grenfell established a seasonal hospital at Indian Harbour in 1894.

His first book, *Vikings of Today*, was published in 1895, and he established the first Co-operative Store at Red Bay and a Mission hospital at Harrington Harbour, Quebec, in 1896. The following year, Grenfell did a lecture tour to Boston and New York, and in 1899, the medical ship *Strathcona* was donated for work on the Labrador.

The years 1900 and 1901 saw the establishment of headquarters at St. Anthony and the organization of Co-operatives at St. Anthony and Flower's Cove. Over the years, up to seven more Co-operatives were established in various places. Grenfell also initiated a sawmill, fox-farm and bait freezer at St. Anthony. An orphanage was opened in St. Anthony in 1906 and an Industrial Department began to sell "Grenfell Crafts" internationally.

In 1907, Grenfell founded a Nursing Station at Forteau, and Grenfell Associations were set up in New York and New England. A reindeer herd and herders were imported to St. Anthony from Lapland, and a non-denominational kindergarten opened in St. Anthony in 1908.

On November 18, 1909, Grenfell married Anne Elizabeth Caldwell MacClanahan of Lake Forest, Chicago, Illinois. Three children were born to them.

The International Grenfell Association was incorporated in 1914, and operated until 1981 when The Grenfell Regional Services Board, a government agency, took it over. The Grenfell connection with the Royal National Mission to Deep Sea Fishermen had ended in 1934. In Labrador, in 2009, medical work is overseen by The Labrador Grenfell Regional Health Authority.

In 1915, Grenfell served with the Harvard Surgical Unit in France, his contribution to the WWI effort. Also, in 1915 the cottage hospital in North West River was established and run by the physician, Dr. Harry Paddon.

The new hospital at St. Anthony was opened on July 25, 1927, and, at this same event, Grenfell was informed that he would be made a Knight Commander of the Ancient Order of Saint Michael and Saint George.

In 1935 he and his wife retired to Vermont. Anne Grenfell died in 1939 and Sir Wilfred Grenfell, M.D., F.R.C.S., K.C.M.G., died on October 9, 1940.

Grenfell was a prolific writer who turned out numerous books and articles. Among them were his first book, *Vikings of Today*, and his first autobiography, *A Labrador Doctor*, published in 1919. Over the years he published thirty-three books, including: *Tales of the Labrador*, *Off the Rocks*, *A Man's Faith*, *A Labrador Logbook*, *The Romance of Labrador*,

The Story of a Labrador Doctor, What Christ Means to Me, Labrador Days: Tales of the Sea Toilers, Adrift on an Ice-pan, Forty Years for Labrador, Down North on the Labrador, Labrador: The Country and the People, Down to the Sea: Yarns From Labrador, Labrador Looks at the Orient, Northern Neighbours: Stories of the Labrador People, and *Labrador and North Newfoundland.*

When Grenfell retired to Vermont in 1935, at the age of seventy, there were in operation, through his efforts, five hospitals, seven nursing stations, two orphanages, fourteen industrial centres, four summer schools, three agricultural stations, twelve clothing distribution centres, several Co-operative Stores, a co-operative lumber mill, and a haul-up slip for ship repairs (Provincial Archives, Government of Newfoundland and Labrador (www.therooms.ca/archives/), "The IGA Magic Lantern Show" (www.iga.nf.net), and Joseph R. Smallwood, ed., *Encyclopedia of Newfoundland and Labrador.* Vol. 2, p. 742).

LETTERS

LOOKING FORWARD TO THE TRIP

Harvard University, Preachers' Room
5 Clunnot Circle
Cambridge, Mass.
July 13th, 1905

My Dearest:

After some preliminary discussion of domestic issues that is irrelevant to the trip, Mr. Moore continues:

Saw Crockett.[3] He says, send letters to W.H. Peters, agt.[4] for Dr. W.T. Grenfell, St. Johns, Newfoundland. But send telegrams to W.T. Grenfell, on board *Strathcona*, Battle Harbor, Labrador. Peters is often able to forward. Crockett says, by no means take watch. So got a dollar one.[5] By all means take a rod for trout. – not so big as my bass rod – fishing magnificent, trout 2 lbs. etc. in all streams. [Told] us what I can do very cheaply. Says boat dirty beyond description.

He will send to ship for use pair of blankets from his sleeping bag. Never warm from start to finish, he says. Food poor. ship staunch, but crank. Grenfell audacious navigator. diseases I read fully prevalent. G's work magnificent. Young Clipston Sturges is up here and will go on cruise.

---

[3] Dr. Crockett, who had gone with Grenfell previously.

[4] agent

[5] Leave your expensive watch at home.

Got your package by express from Portland, almost as soon as I was at house. But nothing yet…from May.[6] Got telegram from Aldrich he will meet me 10:00 a.m. tomorrow at Kirkland St. house. No letters here. Have…one from Summer School. Yet, I shall be pinched for time, C.[7] [this] I know. But must get St. L. paper off, even if the Delano-funeral-paper cannot be finished.

Following some personal comments, Mr. Moore closes:

House so still. and lonely, speaking so much of the days I spent with you here, Hans, Mom and Dorry. This makes lump come in my throat. But it is best to go. I will write you tomorrow. Dearest and deepest love to you and to all.

Your husband,
Edward C. Moore.

PREPARATIONS AND ANXIETIES

5 Clunnot Circle,
Cambridge, Mass.
July 14th

My Darling:

It has been a very hot day. and only now, 8:30, is beginning to rain in a way that may cool the air. No mail was incoming – The office caused its blunder in not giving my note to our carrier until after final delivery. Some will have gone to you. I hope not having to cause you trouble. Forwarding everything to you will be arranged after final delivery tomorrow.

Have telegram from your father about the Bass Rod. but according to

---

[6] Eliza's sister

[7] circa, meaning around

what Crockett said, shd[8] not take it anyway. May's barrel came and was put in cellar, when I was out. I opened top because I did not know what was in it and so how and where to leave it. It seems full of silk [?]…and smells of camphor so I carried it up into the store room…. Had box also containing nursing bag and some stationery.

Here, Mr. Moore discusses in detail the plans he and his wife had for renovating the house in Cambridge. He apologizes for planning to go away at this time and leaving so much work for her; "I cannot bear to leave it all to you to do." He continues:

I saw Kate and told her to wash what few clothes I left in hamper.

Found I could save 8.00 by buying my ticket through to Battle Harbor. Put down 100.00 for first check I took. But it may be advisable to draw 50.00 more tomorrow. Crockett says by all means buy a few furs. So I will if I can for you and May & Dorry. Sweater not finished. But I am to have it at 10:15 tomorrow a.m. Am to make a little speech at Summer School at 10. Have found everything you told me of and begun to pack.

Bought a cheap trout rod etc. Whole thing for 4.50 incl reel, line etc. Got some Listerine, Ponds ex. brandy, chocolate, pads and indelible pencils – and this may… – got a pipe and a can tobacco. It all mounts up. I am sorry. But I will be careful. My ticket cost 27.25 more but it includes meals almost the whole way, viz. a week's board besides transportation, etc.

Leg better. Had your letter. What a day you had of it. So glad Will is [around] with the children. I will telegraph you I think from Battle Harbor when we meet G. unless it costs too much! And now what shall I say. What can I say. I have filled up my letter with all sorts of things. But the real [concern] I cannot miss. How heavy my heart is at going. How wanton and unnecessary and selfish it seems and how happy I was with you and our children at Punkey[9] and how long the silence is going to be! Oh God keep you all and make me worthier of you.

---

[8]   should

[9]   summer vacation place

I go in order that I may come back with verve and talent, that I may make it easier for you. How can I ever speak my gratitude to you for those weeks past, for all the year, and for all the years since we became engaged.

After a personal message Mr. Moore concludes:

Deepest love to you and my children.

Your husband,
Edward C. Moore

JOURNEY TO HALIFAX

Sunday Morning,
July 16th.

My Darling Wife:

Here we are on the most magnificent morning you can imagine. Expecting to be in Halifax by two 0'clock this afternoon and not sailing from there until 6:00 tomorrow morning. We have had a quiet night. Ship spotlessly clean, discipline good, meals excellent. – but not included in ticket as I supposed. Passenger list very full. Countless Nova Scotia servants going home for their vacations. Officers complain that this class have so completely taken possession of their time that few tourists any longer go this way. To my own thinking they are a quiet respectable lot and less objectionable than some tourists I have seen. The officers point of view was probably that they spend less money.

It was very hot in Boston again yesterday. Armstrong was at the house by 7 and caught me in my bath so I had to make haste to get the bag etc. closed up. Got ready for prayers and for my little speech before the Summer School....

Next, Mr. Moore goes into great detail about several events of the previous day and he continues:

Got to the dock at eleven forty five. Bedlam broke loose. Everybody crazy about baggage, and scores to bid each single passenger goodbye. Checked my baggage and went aboard. Sat down to mop my face and read my mail wh[10] I had only partially read going in on the car.... So I know all was well up to that point.

Had nap in afternoon – afternoon rough and vast numbers sick – grief was everywhere – more room to pace deck.... Ship gradually cooled off. Went to bed about 8:30 and dreamed that we were about opposite Portland at that time. Thought lovingly of you and all on little Punkey and then slept until 6:30.

My roommate was a fat, hot, little man going to look at a gold mine forty miles out from Halifax[11] – very important, otherwise very harmless. Calm night and no sea this morning so that the forces are uncovering. I got an extra pair of pyjamas as I could not find the no striped ones. Have they not been torn up?

Here Mr. Moore goes on for 24 pages to write of paying bills, etc., and he shows his concern, once again, for what happens at home while he is away. He continues:

This letter is all taken up with details and is already too long, especially as it is so poorly written. It will not be so much filled up except with new things in the next. But you know how full of love and longing it is.

Crockett gave me a pain when he said that he got all his letters in a batch when he got back to Battle Harbor. But, perhaps, I shall have better luck. Anyway do not think of the trip as one into wh you have urged me. You know how few such things I would ever do unless urged. And yet how I enjoy them afterward and I should never stir

---

[10] which

[11] This gold mine was located in Moose River, Middle Musquodoboit, NS, Halifax County. It was in operation in the late 1800s and early 1900s and open-pit mining was discussed for the same area in 2008 (*The Chronicle Herald*, spring 2008).

from your side and that of the children if I could help it. And yet I doubt if that is best. This certainly is a rare chance.

After more personal comments Mr. Moore concludes:

So grateful to you for what you give me. What you always have given me and been to me. What you are. My wife.

Your husband,
Edward C. Moore

A BRIEF REMINISCENCE

Sunday aft.
July 16th.
In Halifax

Dearest:

Have just been ashore to mail my other letters, and walk about this decayed old town. Thought much of Seth and his service here in Dalhousie College [University] – wh I have seen the outside of – and the death of his beloved Tisha in childbirth here. It was a hard blow to him and to his mother.

Did you get key to silver chest sent by me from Camb.? Did you get box of flowers from Camb. Garden?

21 years ago today that I sailed on the *Enis* to take up my fellowship in Germany.

Dearest love to you and my chicks.

Yours,
E.C.M.

BY TRAIN TO SYDNEY, CAPE BRETON

THE SYDNEY, E. LeRoi Willis, proprietor,
Sydney, C.B., July 18, Tuesday

My Dearest Wife:

I mailed letters Tuesday in Halifax. Had a beautiful run to Hawkesbury[12] and then up the [wide] railway to Sydney first on one side and then on the other of the Bras d'or Lakes. Perfectly beautiful. The place where the train crosses on a bridge from Iona to Grand Narrows is one of the most superb things I ever saw, and I never even so much as heard of it.

I am here for the day to visit Kingman[13] and go aboard the *Bruce*[14] tonight [sailing] to Port aux Basques early tomorrow. Sail on the *Home*[15] tomorrow night from Bay of Islands and expect to be in Battle Harbor Saturday night though the Straits [*sic*] of Belle Isle are full of floating ice. Much of that.

So much does the assortment of ice and cold water that goes through these Straits affect the whole climate of the northern part of the

---

[12] Port Hawkesbury is located in the Strait of Canso between Cape Breton and Nova Scotia.

[13] A medical doctor, a surgeon, who accompanied Moore on this trip with Grenfell.

[14] The S.S. *Bruce* was built in Scotland and arrived in Newfoundland in October 1897 and operated between Little Placentia and North Sydney, NS. After June 30, 1898, the *Bruce* was the first regular ferry between Port aux Basques, Newfoundland, and North Sydney. She was lost in 1911 off Louisbourg, NS, and one or two people drowned (Joseph R. Smallwood, ed., *Encyclopedia of Newfoundland and Labrador*. Vol. 1, p. 279).

[15] The S.S. *Home* was one of the original Newfoundland steamer boats known as the "Alphabet Fleet," i.e., *Argyle, Bruce, Clyde, Dundee, Ethie, Fife, Glencoe,* and *Home*. Later, were added, *Invermore, Kyle, Lintrose,* and *Meagle*. These ferries were part of the service of the Reid Newfoundland Company, 1901 to 1923, created when Robert G. Reid agreed to operate eight subsidized coastal steamers to integrate with the railway around Newfoundland and to connect Newfoundland to Labrador and Nova Scotia. The *Home* served the people on the Labrador until the *Kyle* came into service in 1913. The *Home* sank in Jersey Harbour, NL, in 1952 (Maura Hanrahan, *The Alphabet Fleet*, pp. 137-138).

Dominion that men believe [great] if they cd.[16] close them – only twenty-five miles[17] at the narrowest point and turn the Arctic current over the tip of Newfoundland out into the Gulf Stream that it cd make an absolutely new world here.

This place is so English. So was Halifax. You might have thought yourself in Southampton. Our ship lay at dock from 2:00 Sunday aft. and not a box of freight could be taken out of her until midnight. Then she unloaded in a flash and we sailed at 3:00 a.m.

Red coats everywhere. Salvation Army holding a most successful meeting on the main street. Everybody with a silk hat on, going to Church. The view from the top of the Citadel and over the Harbor is magnificent hardly less so than at Quebec. Here the great interest is an immense steel plant,[18] rails, etc. But Canada is so poor compared with the States.

My leg is all right again, healed over perfectly. Must have got some thing in it that it was so slow in beginning to heal. Erman sent an express package to the *Olivette* of fudge and other sweet [chocolates] to be shared with Grenfell on the *Strathcona*. Was not that very ghim.[19] I had a sweet goodbye note from May too.

Here Mr. Moore instructs his wife that, if certain packages come for him she should not forward them because they might get lost. Also, he has considerable discussion and instructions about the gas and electricity at home, then he continues:

My spirits rise to this [coming trip]. It is going to be a great cruise and a wonderful experience and I mean to get all I can out of it, g[20]

---

[16] could

[17] The <u>Strait</u> of Belle Isle is approximately 125 km long and 15 km wide. Generally known as "The Straits."

[18] The Sydney Steel Corporation (SYSCO), of American investors, established a steel mill in Sydney, NS, in 1901, powered by an abundance of Cape Breton coal. It operated for 100 years under various headings and was sold to a company from India, which began dismantling in 2001. The infamous Sydney Tar Ponds resulted from this mill.

[19] good of him

[20] get

Every kind of good for your dear sake. It is too bad that the Seattle and China trips both come this year. The China one at any rate is impossible. Of course there will be another deputation in four or five years. But it wd. be [prefer]able to go now. I promise I shall decide...

I want to say when the *Home* goes out of the dock tomorrow night I cannot get a letter across the Straits for nearly a week. But you will not worry. I think I will not telegraph before but will reserve that experience until I get to Battle Harbor, on the way out.

Tenderest love, and God keep you, my darling wife. Was it worthwhile that July night, 19 years ago, when you engaged yourself to me? Hug our children for their father.

Your husband,
E.C.M.

ARRIVAL IN NEWFOUNDLAND

Port-aux-Basques,
July 19th. Wednesday

My Darling:

Just arrived, got through custom house[21] and am waiting for the train to start before we can get any breakfast. Had a perfectly still night, much too still for so fine a ship as the *Bruce*. This morning it is dripping with fog, but may burn off later.

Whom should I meet the moment I entered the car but Dr. Alex McKenzie and his son going to Battle Harbor on the *Home*. How much further he is going I do not know. But not on the *Strathcona*[22] I guess. Kingman says he thinks Crockett was wrong in his directions as to mail. Send letters simply, care of Dr. Grenfell, at Battle Harbor, Labrador, for E.C.M. on *Strathcona*. There are two ships from Sydney to one from St. Johns and he thinks the delays will be less. This makes the address for letters same as for telegrams. The others will come. But are subject to more delay. I must get this off, dearest love to you. I miss you so – so much.

Your husband,
Edward.

---

[21] Newfoundland was a country at this time. It became a province of Canada in 1949.

[22] The *Strathcona* was built in Dartmouth, England, in 1899. She was purchased as a medical ship for Grenfell's use on the Labrador, Sir Donald Smith (Lord Strathcona) being the chief donor. He was President of the Hudson Bay Company, the Canadian Pacific Railway, and the Bank of Montreal, and had previously presented the Mission with a ship, *Sir Donald*, for Grenfell's use. The *Strathcona* was eighty feet long and equipped with medical cots, dispensary, and x-ray equipment but had no hold for carrying freight. She was refitted in 1921 but in the late fall of 1923 she sank in a gale of wind off Seldom-Come-By on the Newfoundland coast. There was no loss of life. In 1925, *Strathcona 2* was purchased in Southampton. It is interesting that Harvard University had its own Grenfell Alumni Association, which, one year, undertook to raise money for the expenses of the *Strathcona* (Wilfred Grenfell, *A Labrador Doctor*, p 131 & p. 237).

A BRIEF GREETING

Steamer, *Home*,
Just off from Bay of Islands,
Wednesday aft. July 19th.

My Darling:

The captain says I have just five minutes to get off a note to you from the little Post Office at Birchy Cove, our first landing, and then the letter will go back on the *Bruce* day after tomorrow. Quiet night on the *Bruce*. Magnificent ride on Newfoundland Railway, 145 miles from Port aux Basques to Bay of Islands.

This place is like what I imagine a Norwegian Fiord. Perfectly glorious weather. So well and everything prospering and happy.

Love.
Edward C. Moore.

EXCITEMENT OF A NEW COUNTRY

Bartletts Harbor, Newfoundland,
Thursday Evg. July 20th.

My Dearest:

I have seen so much that is new and strange yesterday and today that unless I get my journal letter started soon I shall forget.

We had not gone five miles out of Port-aux-Basques when we saw great fields of snow lying in the clefts and shadowed places on the mountains. But all about us the flowers were in greatest profusion, buttercups, daisies, great quantities of blue flag, iris in all the marshes, sheep laurel, etc. The road is a narrow gauge one but the train made fair speed[23] and the dining car was especially good. We got off about 9:00 o'clock and were at Bay of Islands about three in the afternoon.

Every here and there the train, which is the only through passenger train in forty-eight hours – there is a freight on alternated days – would stop to let off passengers with rods and guns – let them off I mean at no station but at some place in the wilderness, or to pick up fishermen who had no luck at one stream and wished to be set down at another.[24] We passed no village of more than fifty houses, few of even twenty houses, but all with one and most with two Churches, Catholic and Anglican.

Everywhere in the forests such fearful evidences of fire, acres and even miles burned over, scarcely even a moment when some burned region was not in sight. Such fabulous waste and loss of timber which with the mines and fisheries is the only wealth of the country.

Mountains often 2000 to 2500 feet high, bare and scarred in all their upper portions, often running right down into the sea, and sometimes separated from the sea by a mile or two of low land. Short timber on the low land, but on the mountains often very heavy timber. Skyline often of remarkable beauty owing to the sharp and rugged outlines of the mountains and every here and there the glimpse of the sea. But so few people and those few so poor, so poor. English, Scotch, French, Indians and Esquimaux,[25] a few. A few whale factories, canning establishments, mining plants, and things of that sort.

---

[23] The railway line was completed across Newfoundland in 1897. The first regular express, in 1898, from St. John's to Port aux Basques, took twenty-seven hours and twenty-five minutes to travel the five hundred and forty-eight miles. It was later dubbed "The Newfie Bullet!" (Joseph R. Smallwood, ed., *The Book of Newfoundland*. Vol. 3, pp. 473-502).

[24] This practice was continued during the ninety-year lifespan of the railway, and I have taken advantage of that service to follow good partridge and caribou hunting on the Gaff Topsails in the fall. However, no more, for the last regularly scheduled train made its journey on September 30, 1988.

[25] "Esquimaux" is the French version of "Eskimo" and refers to the aboriginal people who live in Polar regions from Eastern Siberia, across Alaska, Canada, and Greenland. The word was first used by the British Arctic explorer, Samuel Hearn (1745-1792), in his journal, *A Journey from Prince of Wales Fort to the Northern Ocean (1795)*. The term "Esquimaux" is considered offensive today and has been replaced by "Inuit," their language is Inuktitut (Cyril F. Poole, ed., *Encyclopedia of Newfoundland and Labrador*. Vol. 3, pp. 57-65).

Got the little ship, the *Home* at Bay of Islands. Captain a burly capable Englishman named Taylor, wife and baby on board for this trip, lives at Bay of Islands. Sailed shortly after three, and stopped at a half a dozen different places even before dark Carrying mail and the most varied cargo – all passed over the side of the ship into dories wh the Islanders put along side. In many cases very heavy merchandise handled with great skill with some sea running.

Islands numberless. Many of them are remarkably beautiful. On mainland mountains very fine, snow always in sight and often cliffs rising right out of the sea. Moon rose and we went on up the coast in its full splendor. Went to bed early. Rose to find it raining and all day we have alternated fog and rain. But have not been delayed much.

Always this process of putting off and on freight, mails, etc. for this is the one communication of these people with the world and this comes once a week each way in summer only. There are no roads, absolutely none on the mainland, only caribou trails after you get back a few rods from the shore, an almost impassable wilderness, primeval. In the winter they go along the shore flats etc. with a kometick[26] and dogs for then the steamers cannot go.

There are extensive copper mines as at Yorke [York] Harbor and a whale factory as at Hawkes Bay. Lobster canning also at this last place. French man-of-war lying at Yorke Harbor. English man-of-war at Hawkes Bay. Constant friction between the fishermen of the rival interests.

Was much interested in the establishment for trying out whale oil. Whales are towed in – whaling ships from here are all steamers – towed in alongside of ships, drawn up on float, cut up and boiled etc. Every conceivable fragment of him being consumed for some purpose or other. Only a few days ago when the Captain passed down there were two large whales on the float. Of these we now only smelled the smell and saw the vats of fat and oil. I wish we had seen the whales themselves. Saw seals in plenty.

---

[26] The word "komatik" (a type of sled) comes from the Inuktitut language.

Landed also at the cannery for lobsters where the work is so largely done by women – very clean the whole place looked – and it was said to be a very thriving industry and a great variation from the former lives of the women. The English which the people speak strikes me as very noticeably good.

Tonight we are lying here in this Cove for the fog has shut us in. There are countless islands, reefs etc. all about and no light houses anywhere on this coast north of Hawkes Bay. The sense one has of loneliness is one of the dominant impressions. The coast is for the most part absolutely uninhabited. The islands always so, and the sails so few.

The captain met Grenfell last week in Battle Harbour and he told him that he would meet us in Bonne-Esperance[27] on the Labrador Coast and take us off this vessel. If he does that will probably be tomorrow afternoon for Bonne-Esperance is the first point we touch on the Labrador side, we should then go up through the Straits of Belle Isle in his vessel and not in this one, and shd probably spend Sunday at the Hospital at Battle Harbor.

By the way, all this part of Labrador in wh we are to be belongs to Newfoundland and requires 5 (cent) postage.[28] I never knew Labrador was in Newfoundland, politically. But from Blanc Sablon north that is the case.[29] I hope that Grenfells meeting us here

---

[27] A settlement on an island in the mouth of St. Paul's River (formerly Eskimo River), Quebec.

[28] At that time, the Newfoundland five-cent postage stamp (issued 1899 to 1910) was a blue stamp with a portrait of the Duke of York who was to become King George V. In 1941, a postage stamp was issued in memory of Sir Wilfred Grenfell, showing Grenfell on the *Strathcona 2* (Cyril F. Poole, ed., *Encyclopedia of Newfoundland and Labrador*. Vol. 4, p. 415 & p. 422).

[29] In 1763, Labrador was a possession of England. When the English conquered Quebec (Lower Canada), Labrador was placed under the jurisdiction of Newfoundland. In 1774, it reverted to Canada and was returned to Newfoundland in 1809. In 1927 the Judicial Committee of the Privy Council established the western boundary of Labrador at the height of land and confirmed Labrador to be under the authority of Newfoundland. Newfoundland tried to sell Labrador to Canada in 1909 for nine million dollars and again in 1932 for one hundred and ten million. Both joined Canada in 1949 (Tim Borlase, *The Labrador Settlers, Métis and Kablunângajuit*, p. 44f., plus various sources).

does not mean that he is going to the French Shore[30] again. But rather that we shall get right off to the north. I do want to get down to the Moravian Esquimaux Missions anyway. But we shall see.

If we leave the ship tomorrow, I am going to send this by the captain. I must [try to get] some kind of idea where I am going to get a letter and when. But that is perfectly impossible of course. The only thing that one can say is that so long as I have no telegram from you I assume all is well and wait with what patience I can. I cannot even tell about my wife home.

But we have certainly made a remarkably rapid and successful journey down thus far. I have read today during the rain Wallaces account of his journey with Hubbard. *The Lure of the Labrador Wild*,[31] in which journey Hubbard lost his life. Such a foolish sacrifice.

It does not seem possible that it is only a week today that I said goodbye to you at Punkey and in Portland. It seems so far away, and it was all so dear and happy. God bless and keep you all.

Your Husband.
Edward.

---

[30] By the Treaty of Utrecht (1713), the French could fish on the Newfoundland coast between Cape Bonavista on the east coast around to Point Riche on the northwest coast. The Treaty of Versailles (1783) changed the boundaries to include the shore between Cape St. John on the northeast coast to Cape Ray on the southwest coast. There seemed to be a continual dispute about fishing rights around this coast. Moore obviously meant by the "French Shore" the area around St. Anthony and the northern tip of the island (Joseph R. Smallwood, ed., *Encyclopedia of Newfoundland and Labrador*. Vol. 2, pp. 407-415).

[31] Leonidas Hubbard, an American, undertook a Labrador expedition in 1903, along with Dillon Wallace and guide George Elson. They planned to go from North West River to Ungava Bay but took the wrong river; their canoes overturned and they never reached their destination. After they turned back, Hubbard died of starvation before reaching supplies. In 1905, at the same time Moore was in Labrador, Hubbard's widow, Mina, completed the journey (Dillon Wallace, *The Lure of the Labrador Wild*).

ACROSS THE STRAIT OF BELLE ISLE

S.S. *Home*,
Off Blanc Sablon, Coast of Labrador,
Friday, July 21st.

My Dearest Wife:

We stayed last night at Bartletts Cove[32] because of the dense fog, but were off this morning at 3:00 oclock with the first light, have called at two of these isolated little ports and put off cargo, mail and passengers. And now we are headed directly across the Straits for Blanc Sablon and just to the west of that is Bonne-Esperance where we are to meet Grenfell. That will probably be before dark tonight.

We have had the first heavy sea of the trip and the ship is light so that she rolls a good deal. There have been intervals when the fog lifted though it has been gray all day, and in the first of these clear periods just after we left Flower[33] Cove, we saw fourteen ice-bergs of varying sizes, some low, and one as high as the masts of a schooner which was passing near it. The captain says he never saw so many so far west in the Straits, and of course this accounts for the fog and may retard our progress and Grenfells, too. I have been using your glass all morning and am a thousand times grateful to you for it. It is splendid.

The icebergs are fine. So blue and clean as if they came from a land where dust, and mud and soot were never known. I imagine our passage eastward down the Straits tomorrow will be through a procession of them. We on Grenfells boat, will probably keep in close to the Labrador shore. But today in crossing we have been in the course of the Montreal and Quebec transatlantic liners, who will hardly expect ice bergs so far west. We passed within a quarter of a mile of one wh the captain estimated to be at least 120 feet high at its highest end.

---

[32] Bartletts Harbour

[33] Flower's Cove

I hate to leave the *Home*. She has been most comfortable and cozy and is most seaworthy.

Kingman and I have left word with the Captain that we want rooms on his trip out from Battle Harbor Sunday Sept 3, as it may be before he gets away. This is safer as there will be a rush westward at that time. If after talking with Grenfell he confirms this I shall write to the purser of the *Bruce* and to this office of the Intercolonial Boat, to arrange passage all the way.

The eclipse[34] is on Wed. the 30th, and G. is to be at Indian Harbor. It ought to be easy to get to Battle Harbor by the 2nd, then in Bay of Islands on the 5th and get the *Bruce* that night from Port aux Basques be in Sydney Thursday a.m. early and…in Boston Friday a.m. your birthday. This will be the earliest possible. If I come down by [train] either to Boston or New York, and especially if I go back by St. Johns it will be two or three days later. I am thinking that by that time, I shall want to get to you as quickly as possible. That Friday the 8th is seven weeks from today and one week is already gone since I left you.

I can but think how you would enjoy all this. It is so strange and beautiful. This goes with my dearest love.

Your husband,
Edward.

---

[34] A total solar eclipse was experienced in Labrador on August 30, 1905, at 13:07 hours. The umbral shadow in North America had a width of one hundred and ninety-two kilometres so that the geographic region around Cartwright, Indian Harbour, North West River, etc., experienced a total eclipse for three minutes and forty-six seconds. People came to this area from far and near to be in an advantageous position for viewing this event (www.sciencemag.org).

FIRST IMPRESSIONS OF LABRADOR

S.S. *Home,*
Off Lance au Loup, Coast of Labrador,
Saturday, July 22nd.

My Dearest:

We got into Bonne-Esperance last night about 5:00 oclock only to find that the *Strathcona* had been there and gone, taking her mail but leaving no word as to where she was going. We made our station Salmon Cove and then went back to Bonne-Esperance because it seemed as if in the dense fog we should have to spend the night there. Later, it lifted and we got away. It came down again after we went to bed and the Captain anchored off the fog horn and light at Blanc Sablon, not daring to try to go in.

This morning when the light came we saw a large schooner hard and fast on the rocks, all sails set. Had gone on during the night, and the man-of-war, lying in the harbor, the *Scylla*, was sending two boats crews to see if they could not help her get off.

This is quite a place, a big whale factory, a Russian barque unloading coal, two sealing steamers in port. We have had but momentary glimpses of the region back of the immediate shores. But as yet have not seen a single tree. Only low stunted stuff. But the cliffs are very fine red granite, for the most part, with green grass in the crevices, just now in the midst of the short summer. Stratification almost horizontal in most cases. Deep water almost up to shore in most places. But quite the contrary at Blanc Sablon, there countless little islands and many dangerous reefs.

Have seen at least a hundred ice bergs, one of them hard aground in 180 feet of water. So you can imagine the size. The thermometer is about 48, and the barometer low. Heavy fog all the time. The

Captain says he never saw so much ice so far to the west and rarely ever made a foggier trip. But we are not so much behind his time table, though we shall not get into Battle Harbor until tomorrow, Sunday, morning.

Of course we may pick up Grenfell at any port from here onward. But the Captain thinks it possible that he over-estimated the delay the fog would cost us and crossed the Straits from Bonne-Esperance to Flower Cove, passing us on the way. In that case he will have to follow us to Battle Harbor where we shall wait for him. Incidentally, one learns that he has the reputation of being the most impatient and irresponsible of navigators, doing things which no one up here dreams of doing.

The men look so old. Even those whom you know to be young. The life is so hard. They are good humored, but very silent – reticence itself, rarely speaking but in monosyllables and with difficulty projecting themselves into the position of your ignorance of that wh they know so well. Huge big boats, like a man-of-war's boats. Dories almost as big, oars are like sweeps, 20 and 24 feet long, having a peg, like a thole pin,[35] stuck through the oar about a foot from the handle to aid the men in turning the oar back and forth when sculling.– wh they do very much. Sails almost always dyed dark red or dark brown with bark of trees so as to keep them from rotting.

Cod fishing has been poor. Whales few and wild. Seals very plentiful. Boots and moccasins are made of their soft-tanned hides and fat used to adulterate cod liver oil.

Great cascades on the shore plunging down the bluffs into the sea. Snow everywhere, sometimes within a few rods of the villages. Water always black under this fog. I presume it wd. be very different under bright sunlight. Rumors that the ice is such that we cannot get to Battle Harbor. But I do not believe that. But I am afraid that the ice

---

[35] A wooden peg set in the gunwale of a boat for holding the oar while rowing.

is such that the whole shore will be swathed in fog for two weeks yet, and navigation be difficult.

To think that it is not yet even a week since I left Boston in such sweltering heat. Oh how I long to know how you and my dear children are.

Kingman already has a good many fine photographs. I am going to pay for part developing when he gets back and so am in for a goodly share. He is not a very big man – has come up from the ranks – is rather opinionated and of great self esteem but means well and my particular angles do not need to run against his. He defends Duncan.[36] Believes in the newspapers etc. in a way that I do not.

Have necessarily seen a good deal of the McKenzies. The son is very much like the mother in this that it is very difficult to tell what he is like. Father very much spoiled by attention in times past and pitifully wanting it now. Painfully old every way and clearly not at all aware of it or willing to concede it. They are in a stew lest the *Portia*[37] may sail for St. Johns without them, today or tomorrow. It has been hard to keep off professional and environmental questions in a way I did not think good for the other man. More tomorrow. Most devoted love, my darling.

Your husband, Edward.

---

[36] Norman Duncan published *Doctor Luke of the Labrador* the previous year.

[37] The *Portia* was a Bowring Brothers vessel which was subsidized by the government of Sir Robert Bond in 1904 for the service from St. John's to St. Anthony. She was used until retired in 1940 (Cyril F. Poole, ed., *Encyclopedia of Newfoundland and Labrador*. Vol. 4. p. 403).

MEETING UP WITH GRENFELL

Battle Harbor,
The Newfoundland Labrador,
July 24th.

My Dearest Wife:

I wrote you three letters mailed from Halifax and one mailed from North Sydney. Then there was a little note sent back from Port-aux-Basques, and two more sent back by the *Home* to be mailed today in Bay of Islands. This, therefore is letter eight. And then I telegraphed you from Chateau, twenty-five miles west of here, because I learned to my chagrin that there is no telegraph connection at all east of Chateau...Indian Harbor but the gap between here and Chateau is fatal. It is a quarrel between the Canadian and the Newfoundland governments and is not going to be made up at once.[38] You can do nothing but telegraph, as I have always said, to Grenfells care here at Battle Harbor. It will come to Chateau by wire and then be sent here on the next boat and forwarded north by semaphore on the wireless. But I hope there will be no need.

We could not understand why the *Strathcona* kept on about an hour and a half ahead of us all down the coast. But when we got here we solved it. He had a French woman on board whom he was bringing

---

[38] The Anglo-American Telegraph Company had a fifty-year monopoly, which expired in 1904 when the telegraph system became Newfoundland Postal Telegraphs, a sub-department of the General Post Office ("Communication in Newfoundland" by J. T. Meaney. In Joseph R. Smallwood, ed., *The Book of Newfoundland*. Vol. 1, pp. 328-338). In the summer of 1904, the Marconi Company built stations at Battle Harbour, Venison Island, Domino, American Tickle, and Smokey in Labrador. In 1906, the operation of these stations for the Newfoundland government was taken over by the Marconi Wireless Telegraph Company of Canada, Ltd., and the facilities were greatly extended and much new equipment was added. In 1910, stations were built at Holton, Cape Harrison and Makkovik. It seems that Moore came to Labrador at a time when negotiations about telegraph communication were proceeding and it was a year later before better communications were available ("The Story of Marconi in Newfoundland" by J. J. Collins. In Joseph R. Smallwood, ed., *The Book of Newfoundland*. Vol. 2. pp. 442-444).

up from Whale Head, 200 miles west, to be operated on. She had a tumor which Kingman and Grenfell and Simpson removed this morning and which weighed 87 pounds, more than the little woman weighs now that it has been removed. She is 37 years old, left 7 little children on the shore down there. Her husband came along with her and has been pacing the walk in dumb agony all day. The present prospect is good that she will pull through. But I am running ahead of my story.

We got to Cape Charles, three miles away at dark and the fog was so dense we did not dare to come over. Lay at Cape Charles all Saturday night and were landed with the first streaks of light, viz., about 3:40 a.m. yesterday, Sunday.

Dr. McKenzie and his son were in a dreadful stew for fear they would not get the *Portia* back to the French coast of Newfoundland and so to St. Johns. But in fact they did not leave until this morning – somewhat to everybody's relief…

We came up to the hospital. There was the Inscription all across the front in the wooden letters which the Cambridge boys had made, Inasmuch as ye have done it unto one the least of these[39] etc. This was of two years ago. The one made last year was for Indian Harbor. Their wood was not heavy enough and already it is beginning to go to pieces.

It was a glorious morning, the finest of this year thus far they all say, sky and sea so blue, forty or fifty big ice bergs in sight. Thermometer just above freezing.

Our landing, or rather the whistle of steamer when she came in set every Esquimaux dog[40] in Battle Harbor howling. The howl is unlike anything I ever heard, long, musical cry. But it gets on one's nerves.

---

[39] Inasmuch as ye have done it unto one of the least of these my brethren, ye have done it unto me" (St. Matthew 25:40b, Bible, King James Version).

[40] Moore's reference here is to the Labrador Husky dog which is of mixed northern breeds and akin to the wolf. They are sled dogs accustomed to hauling heavy loads and are sometimes vicious fighters. On average, a husky dog is between 24-27 inches high and weighs between 50-80 pounds (www.explorelabrador.nf.ca).

And the beasts are so big and have such evil faces and such evil reputations. They will pull down a man from behind just like a pack of wolves. No cow, or horse, no sheep or goat, could live here a moment without being watched all the time by a man. To shut them up in a pen would be nothing. The dogs will pull any pen to pieces.

Simpson and Mrs. Simpson soon came down. Simpson is the dr. who wrote Hans such a nice letter. Mrs. Simpson was a nurse. Both were long at Indian Harbor. Both very English. He a Congregationalist, very 'Moodyish' and Evangelical. But Grenfell is that, too, tho[41] a Ch. of England man.[42]

Kingman and I were shown up to a room hung full of pelts and skins of foxes, otters and lynxes, some very beautiful ones which I am going to price when Simpson gets time.

We washed and dressed and took a long walk – the island is so little, only a few times as big as Punkey villages, opposite harbor full of boats, no fishing done on Sunday, though this is the height of season and the catching time is so short, only two or three weeks, and the catch this year has been so poor.

The *Strathcona* lay in harbor, but we did not see Grenfell until after breakfast. Had the most characteristic English breakfast. Bacon and eggs and toast & tea, after porridge, though eggs have to come from St. Johns. Not a hen in all this part of the world any more than a cow or a pig, and for the same reason. Had prayers before breakfast.

House is full of Mildmay Calendars and texts. Pleasant, comfortable house. Some books – medical and religious. Heated by coal in the main though wood is also used. Natives use wood altogether and use as little as possible because they have to bring it in boats from so far inland. They stack it as Indians would stack wigwam poles, to keep it from getting too wet and soggy and to be able to find it in the deep snows.

---

[41]   although

[42]   In 1885, his second year at university in London, Grenfell attended an evangelistic tent meeting led by the American evangelist, Dwight L. Moody. Grenfell acknowledged that this meeting had a powerful effect on his whole life.

The thermometer rarely goes below than thirty or forty below zero, but there is almost constant high winds and the winter lasts from mid-September till mid-June, sometimes. Snow is visible everywhere here now, though we see no rocks more than a few hundred feet high. I counted 72 ice bergs in sight before we came in to breakfast. But there is no sheet or floe ice such as was reported.

McKenzie preached in the morning and I in the afternoon. McKenzie again in the evening when it became apparent that he was going to stay over. Grenfell read the service all three times. Little Church so quaint and touching, but with some effort to be beautiful in a very simple way, holds about 200 – full three times – people from other islands and men from the fleet in the harbor, some of them. Graves in yard so pathetic, tombstone of little Prince Pomiuk,[43] so many young people, both men and women, both in the church and for that matter in the graveyard to judge by the stones. But all the evidences of a hard, hard life. English people they are here, almost entirely, few French, or Irish or Scotch, no Indians or Esquimaux.

Hardly any flowers except pink heather and the little white flower of the bake-apple berry. Have not seen a tree since mid way up Newfoundland coast. Is no soil here properly speaking, only peat, rotten roots, moss etc. quaking at every foot step and soggy with water. Every hole is at once a pool. But in winter all must be frozen hard as iron.

As it drew towards dark while McKenzie preached last night, I thought of an evening hour when I kneeled beside you far up the Alps in the little chapel at Tiefenkasten. On the way up to Pontresima. Just the same biting air, just the same rugged homely place, just the same devout poor – these are all Protestants as those were Catholics. McK. seemed so old and feeble, leaned on things was so unkempt

---

[43] Pomiuk was the name of an Inuit boy at the "Eskimo Village" located outside the fairgrounds of the World's Fair in Chicago in 1893. He was the son of a northern Inuit chieftain called Kaiachououk. His Christian name was Gabriel and he was about ten years old in 1893. Gabriel Pomiuk fell and broke his hip and never completely recovered. After the exhibition ended, the Inuit were sent back to Labrador where Pomiuk died at the hospital in Battle Harbour. He became well known through Grenfell's writings (Wilfred Grenfell, *A Labrador Doctor*, pp.162-164).

and sloppy, and spoke so characteristically. Grenfell, I think however thought it fine.

I have had a good talk on trip with Wood, the agent of the Deep Sea Fishermen Mission Society[44] from London who is out here to see the work. He sees Grenfells strong points but I think finds him hard to work with and says his subordinates find it hard to work under him. He has so little head for detail and is so unaccountable in his movements. And [with this] Wood feels some danger that the 'Grenfell Assertiveness,' etc. in the U.S. may be building up the work too much on the personal basis and that it may be very difficult for them to plan for it with G.[45]

Took tea on board the *Strathcona* with G. and saw all our arrangements for the next few weeks. Sturges of Boston, a boy about 21 who has been in Harvard, very fat and I judge lazy, is on board and then an individual named Jones who acts as G's secretary, then there are seven in the crew. The skipper seems a fine sort of man.[46]

Kingman was a good deal disturbed because surgical and photographic stuff which he had sent north by Peters in St. Johns, in the middle of May, is not here though he wrote to Peters and as well to Grenfell to see to them. I say one box. But only one of four seems to be on hand. It is rather trying. The auxiliary boat, a schooner, the *Blake* is lying here, too, and Kingman and I, besides Grenfell and Simpson, and Sturges & Jones, searched both her hold and the store house on the dock for two hours, all in vain.

Such confusion in the house on the dock you never saw. Boxes for G. and the mission from everywhere in New England, marked to

---

[44] The Royal National Mission to Deep Sea Fishermen was established in 1884 especially to serve fishermen in the North Sea. This British, evangelical, medical mission employed Grenfell first to serve the North Sea, then, in 1892, it supported him in his work in Labrador until 1934 when the International Grenfell Association (incorporated in 1914) assumed responsibility (www.iga.nf.net).

[45] Grenfell

[46] Moore later refers to him as Captain Bartlett. He is one of the renowned Bartletts of Brigus, Newfoundland. Possibly, he was Captain William Bartlett, father of Captain Bob Bartlett of Arctic exploration fame.

contain books, clothing, machinery, medical, photographic stuff, supplies of every sort, received any time within the last six weeks – some which Simpson thinks came last year. Many more with no mark to indicate their contents, most of wh. have never been opened and piled in there mountains high.

A shipload of stuff. And nobody knows what it is or when it will be got at. In the fall I suppose when the rush of the short season is over. But then it will be too late to use many of the things or at least too late to use them this year. I have not given G. Mays bag or Dorotheas stockings or Hans magazine as yet. I will when we go aboard this afternoon.

Thus far, G.'s mind has been full of the case and of bossing the job of getting the foundations laid for a new doctor's house here at Battle Harbor. Wood leaves the ship here. We all expect if the woman does well to go aboard – i.e. all but Simpson, of course – this afternoon and steam down to St. Anthony, on the Newfoundland shore where G. has a half dozen patients for K.[47] – whom, by the way, I have been all wrong in describing as occulist. He is a surgeon. Whose specialty has been abdominal crisis and particularly…

We shall be back here by the end of the week and then start for Indian Harbor and so on to Hamilton Inlet, to Nain and the Moravian settlements. This will give me the chance to get some mail here at the end of…trip of the *Home*. So only my mistake in having you send letters to St. Johns, instead of here direct, does not favor my getting any at all. I am wondering if mother is with you, if you are going to be at Punkey this coming week and what you and Hans are then going to do when Dorothea goes to mothers. I do not know what to do but to send my letters to Cambridge. Dearest love and much thought and prayer that you all may be kept as well as I have been.

Your husband.
Edward.

---

[47] Kingman

ACCOMPANYING GRENFELL ON MEDICAL VISITATIONS

S.S. *Strathcona*,
Cape Norman, Newfoundland
Wed. Evg. July 26th.

My Dearest:

I wrote you on Monday at noon from Battle Harbor. We thought the *Virginia Lake*,[48] the mail boat, bound for St. Johns, might come in at any time. Wood and I worked hard in the effort to bring some sort of order out of the confusion of the store house on the dock. Two or three new cases for operation had come in, and the French woman's case was very precarious. It was decided not to sail until next day at midday and debated if Kingman should not stay at Battle while Grenfell with the *Strathcona* shd. go back along the east coast of Newfoundland as far as St. Anthony, visit some places wh. otherwise he would not see this year, and bring up some three or four women to Battle Harbor for operation, and this was finally accepted as the plan.

Wood and I spent another morning in the store house, this time also opening boxes and sorting contents etc. Almost the last box which I opened was one from Providence wh. when I opened I found to be from Miss Martha Talbot and including a little wooden box of xmas gifts from the Ministering Childrens League of the Central Cong. Ch. There were notes from both Miss Talbot and Mrs. Barrows. All the clothing so fine and soft and exquisitely packed and the little box so dainty and sweet and Christmas like. So characteristic of the Central Ch. and Miss Talbot and Mrs. Barrows and so unlike so many of the boxes I had been opening.

I cannot [thank you enough], for it was you who opened up this work to that Church. And the things and the whole aim of it made me so

---

48 The *Conscript*, built in 1882, was a steamer employed by Harvey & Co. on the northern service, i.e., St. John's to St. Anthony and along the Labrador coast. In 1891, the *Conscript* was renamed the *Virginia Lake* and continued to be used on that route. She also went to the "Front" as a sealing vessel from 1902 to 1909 when she caught fire and sank while at the ice (Cyril F. Poole, ed., *Encyclopedia of Newfoundland and Labrador*. Vol. 5, p. 488).

happy and so home sick. I fairly fondled each one. And I left full explanations with Mrs. Simpson so there should be no mistakes.

We sailed at 2:00 p.m. Kingman staying behind, somewhat grouchy, as if Grenfell was not paying him attention enough, and I admired Grenfells…decision. It seems that the Governor of Newfoundland[49] comes to Chateau next Saturday and Grenfell is very anxious to see him before starting north as it may result in his getting a few light houses and things he has been fighting for for years. And that is another reason why we should not start north until after this week.

The boat is – oh, so tiny for the things she sets out to do, the storms she meets, distances she cruises, numbers of people and masses of things she carries. And she is in confusion both on decks and below decks because G. does not really mind it and because his assistants are most of them so very inefficient. She is however not so dirty as Crockett led us to think – sufficiently dirty however – And conveniences for washing etc. most rudimentary. I have a room to myself until we pick up Kingman again, and after that it will be crowded enough. G. has his own little cabin but it is dispensary as well.

The fat boy from Boston, Sturges is…on G. of the worst sort. So lazy and inefficient, nominally hospital assistant – but really simply taking the place wh. might be filled by an efficient man. It is just so with the secretary, a y.m.c.a. young man from Toronto whose earlier life has not been just straight. But whose parents, when he confessed conversion, were anxious to propel him into mission work. And Grenfell took him, for his – Jones'– sake rather than for the help which he himself so much needs. It is too bad [he cannot take another man] on or G's work will suffer.

A funny old white haired Englishman for cook who delights to say, "we seamen," though I doubt if he has ever been outside of the galley. A skipper much tried by G's unaccountable doings and the uncertainties wh. attend all his movements. Two engineers and two seamen beside a cabin boy. Two grown dogs, a collie and a retriever, three pups, two of which are the retriever's own and one an

---

[49] His Excellency, Sir William McGregor, M.D., K.C.M.G.

Esquimaux komatik dog wh she is willing to suckle with her own and three little fox pups for the fox-farm[50] wh G. picked up a few days back from a schooner. They had been put in a blubber-cask and their coats are still very sticky. But they play with the pups and are very tame and very amusing.

This menagerie is all over the deck, falls down the companionway, is always having its feet or its tail trodden upon and yelping for pain when not yelling for food. The food – ours, I mean, and the pups and foxes largely partake of our own – is not nearly so bad as I was led to think. The boiled canned beef is pretty bad but we have had a fresh salmon and today bought a lamb and got fresh milk. And the canned things and very good tongue, vegetables and the like, soups etc.

It is as cold as Greenland. Everywhere ice and snow. But I have not felt it in any way. The smells on the cod-schooners and on the wharfs and splitting and drying stages when we land are the worst. They more nearly lay me out than anything which we have yet met. And the closeness and foul air of the fishermens houses is, if possible, worse.

We crossed the Straits in a straight line past the western end of Belle Isle and spent the night at Onion Bay. The fishermen swarm aboard almost so soon as the anchor is down, and seem so glad to see Grenfell. Poisoned hands are the commonest things among these men just now, teeth to be pulled out, 'bad stomachs,' which the condition of their teeth go far to account for, 'fog-eye,' from the dense fogs of these last few weeks, many, many cases of ulcer about mouths, lips, tongues. One man had fallen down a hatch and cracked his ribs. Many cases of skin disease, scurvy and another wh I will not name, all showing poor food, etc. These are the men who come aboard.

It was almost nine before we could get clear to go ashore and visit two houses from which emissaries had come out. One was the case

---

[50] This was Grenfell's first attempt at starting a fox-farm at St. Anthony. He says that he had no time or money to carry on the work and had no success with breeding the foxes. The effort was discontinued when P.E.I. began fox-breeding around 1913 (Wilfred Grenfell, *A Labrador Doctor*, p. 158f).

of a dropsical old man, who had twelve children. Two sons and three daughters were at home, from say 30 down to 15. The two sons were running the business 'trapping'[51] for cod and had five 'share-men' [52] from up the coast to help them. All were sitting with the family in the one large room, men all smoking and spitting incessantly on the floor, one snoring in the corner. Much impressed with the conduct of the girls, so proper and worthy.

Grenfell, after he had seen the old man in next room, asked me to hold prayers. All knelt – one of girls was reading Bible when we came in – all joined in the Lords Pr. I wondered if you cd. have done that just in that way at Gloucester. It is pure English stock, almost no admixture, and so God fearing and upright. With so little opportunity, anyway. Of course there are scoffers. But not many, and few indifferent.

The other visit of that evening was to a married daughter of this same old man who will have to go to the St. Anthony Hospital in the fall, when she is able, just now she has a child two weeks old and cannot go. Such a tale of suffering. And in this house the inhabitants could have been counted by millions and we stood in the middle of the room for precaution.

This morning when we cd. get away, steamed over to Ha Ha Bay, went through the same sort of routine. While G. was doing the sailors on deck, I went with the skipper, Sturges and a man to get a cord of wood for the engines wh was stacked up on the shore for us and by wh. G. hoped to save coal. Landed at low tide through what I took to be roughly a hundred thousand cod heads etc. and whatever else I may forget of all that befalls me, I shall never forget that odour.

The bay was full of schooners and most of them were doing quite fairly well. They estimate their catch by the quantity wh will give a

---

51 This involved the use of the cod-trap as opposed to the seine, hook-and-line, jigger or trawl.

52 Traditionally, on the Labrador, each crew was employed by a "skipper" and given food and lodging. At the end of the season fifty percent of the total catch went toward expenses and the remaining fifty percent was divided equally among the crew members, including the skipper.

quintal, or 112 lbs when it is dried and cured. So when a man says he has got a hundred quintals thus far this season you can think what a mountain of raw fish that means, brought in each night and promptly cleaned, split salted etc. They pitch them out of their dories unto decks or stages with pitchforks[53] and burn great fagots[54] behind a tarpaulin to shield them from the wind when they have to split far into the night. It is a weird scene.

We went down this afternoon to call on an old man named Parmenter, who is now 70 years old, was born at Conception Bay, but his father came from Southampton, Eng. This man, with his wife and baby, fishing for seals, thirty-six years ago, lost his schooner and all of his crew on this head land. But he was able to save wife and baby, and tools and food enough to get them through the winter. Built a 'tilt' wh. has grown into quite a decent house. It was nine months before a human being knew they were here. By that time they were not eager to get away, and here they are still. Twenty odd years ago they buried five children on one day from diphtheria. Here, too, three 'share-men' of the son were sitting in the kitchen, and here, too, we held prayers with resounding 'amens.'

A poor woman who was brought aboard tonight, and whom we shall pick up later and take to the hospital at Battle Harbor for Kingman to operate upon, said she had hoped ever since last October that the Doctor would not fail to run into this cove this summer as she needed to see him so and thought she might die if another year had to go round. How it will be if we get three or four sick women in the little Hospital Room on board and then have rough weather I do not know. Thus far, it has been uncommonly smooth. One sighs for some wind to drive away the fog.

Grenfell was so glad to get Mays nursing bag, and was profuse in his thanks wh. he bids me send and he will send later. He was delighted, too, with Hans' beautiful magazine. It lies here in the cabin now and

---

[53] prongs

[54] A fagot is a bundle of sticks tied together for fuel to create a torch. In Newfoundland and Labrador it also meant a stack of cod-fish in the process of drying.

everybody praises its beautiful pictures etc. It will be left at the St. Anthony Hospital. Dorothea's pair of knitted socks, he has promised to pick out a little girl and let me give them to her myself and take her name and family history. Just now they are in my bag and I fondle them every day for her dear sake.

A Russian Jew peddler has been just ahead of us imposing on the people outrageously. They took him in in their houses as they do everybody. There are no hotels and he utilizes the occasion to palm off on them his worthless stuff at exorbitant prices. He sold to a man at Onion Bay a nickel watch and brass chain for silver and gold at 21.00 wh I do not think are worth 3.00. Grenfell took affidavits and got out a process and proposes at Griquet to haul him on board and try him in his own capacity as magistrate.[55] He has the watch and is warning everybody, means to give him the grand bounce from the shore if he can get hands on him. He also has a liquor-place near St. Anthony which he means to raid. So we are not likely to lack for employment.

Heard a long story from a dear old man at Cape Norman this morning – Thursday – about the vicious rivalry of the Ch. of England people and the Methodists. Here are two Churches to the 20 houses. Ch. of England people, on Grenfell's own testimony, the worst sinners of all. No services of either but once in three months, when either emissary spends most of his time advising the people not to go to the other.

But the thing comes out at its worst in the school. There the Ch. of England teacher beats the Methodist children violently, and holds them up to ridicule. Grenfell himself says the feud is the reason why

---

[55] "A Directory of Magistrates and Justices of the Peace" lists Arthur Squarey as District Magistrate in the St. Anthony District and lists Sir Wilfred T. Grenfell, M.D., K.C. M.G., Mark Alcock, and Noah Simms as Justices of the Peace. In *A Labrador Doctor*, Grenfell refers to himself in one instance as Magistrate and in another as Justice of the Peace. It appears that on the coast of Labrador there was some overlap in the work of both (Joseph R. Smallwood, ed., *The Book of Newfoundland.* Vol. 2. pp. 311-313). In one instance, in his capacity as magistrate, when dealing with five poachers of some animals from his reindeer herd, Grenfell wrote, "I had to be owner, complainant, judge and jailer all rolled into one" (Wilfred Grenfell, *A Labrador Doctor*, p. 211).

no Co-operative store[56] can be planted here and yet through them being at the mercy of the traders they are at this moment practically without salt and the fish they catch after a day or two will rot on their hands. The Bishop[57] is behind it all. This must go off at St. Anthony. Dearest love.

Your husband.
Edward.

A PERSONAL LETTER

Strathcona,
St. Anthony, Newfoundland,
Friday, July 28th.

My Dearest Wife:

We will not count this letter as one of the series. I have written the others as a sort of running journal. And I do not know if it is interesting to you. But it is the only way to preserve a sort of recollection of all these new impressions. And I am afraid all my letters must go in a bundle so that it will be more than you care to read when you get them thus all at once. But this is not to be a journal but just a letter for our engagement day.

My room is none too pleasant when I have it to myself. But now that the poor woman is in the hospital the secretary, Jones, has to room with me and I stay out of my room all that I can. And I have been up

---

[56] In 1896, Grenfell established a Co-operative store in Red Bay, on the Labrador coast. Then, in 1900-01, Co-operatives were set up at St. Anthony and Flower's Cove on the Newfoundland coast. Other Co-operatives followed at West St. Modeste, Great Brehat, Cape Charles, Ragged Islands, Battle Harbour, and, possibly, a couple of other places ("Labrador's Fight for Economic Freedom" by S. W. Grenfell. In Joseph R. Smallwood, ed., *The Book of Newfoundland.* Vol. 6, pp. 346-356 and various other sources).

[57] The Rt. Rev. Llewelyn Jones, 1840-1918, was the fourth Bishop of the Anglican Diocese of Newfoundland and Bermuda from 1878 to 1917.

stairs walking the deck and thinking and remembering and I will write you a letter now here in the cabin before I go to bed. It is odd to think that the letter cannot start until the *Home* next Saturday – a week tomorrow – from Battle Harbor.

There follows a long personal letter and Mr. Moore concludes:

I am thinking of this and trying to be able to recall some delightful and some very pathetic stories of the life and people of this place. It is such a world by itself so remote, so full of character of its own, so fouly represented by Duncan or by any one who has yet written about it. But this letter was just for you.

Your husband,
E.C.M.

BUSY ON THE *STRATHCONA*

Strathcona,
St. Anthony,
July 28th.

My Dearest:

Yesterday afternoon, after I wrote, we ran into Fortune Bay[58] to try to catch the Jew. But he had gone. So G. left the process and testimony with an old magistrate there and went on his way. He cannot take the time now to follow it up. But he thinks the magistrate wd. like nothing better.

As we went out, we met a boat in which were two men and two women and presently we saw that one of the women held a baby. They had rowed out seven miles in a stiff breeze and a lumpy sea because the baby was ill. We slowed down, took them all aboard – over our ten cords of wood strewed everywhere on the

---

[58] A settlement, named Fortune, was located near Griquet, north of St. Anthony.

decks wh. G. is taking down for a poor widow with four children at St. Anthony – examined the baby, prescribed – incidentally – for the woman, too, and put them off again for their row home.

Later, we ran into Karpon bay[59] just to leave word with her husband about one of the women operated on at Battle Harbor Monday. To save time, G. put off in an Esquimaux Cayak [kayak], which he has had lying on the top of the wheel house. It is but little wider or heavier than a shell, made of birch, covered with raw seal hide, stretched and sewed, and is rowed with a two ended paddle not more than three fingers wide. G. was very expert with it. Later, we put off in the dory to pick up some ice of the floating stuff from one of the bergs. We passed a great berg with a hole through it, arch like. But we were too far off to get any pictures of it.

In St. Leonard's[60] Bay, I went off with G. to see the wife of a fisherman who had 14 children, 12 of them at home. The woman was pretty sick and the man has taken but a few fish this season – 'this voyage,' – as they call it, – meaning this season. Even when they sleep on land every night – So the prospect is for a pretty miserable winter.

They are English people named Colburne, and to one of his children, Deborah, I gave Dorothea's stockings, and then when the man in his gratitude pressed upon Grenfell a little snow-white seal skin, beautifully cured, Grenfell gave it to me and told me to take it to Dorothea and establish connection with the household here. The white seal skins are from the baby seals killed or captured with their mothers in the sealing season. This little animal can hardly have been a foot and a half long. I know Dorothea will be delighted to have it for the floor of her little room.

This morning early we ran into St. Anthony and landed the wood and all of Grenfell's boxes and stuff wh. had been accumulating at Battle Harbor. And have just been out to the headland again to tow out a schooner laden with salt for the relief of the fishermen farther

---

[59] Quirpon

[60] St. Lunaire

north. She was held here by the calm and could not get out. While the salt is very much needed over there.

I am going up after dinner to visit the hospital and school and orphanage with Grenfell and he has very much on his mind, a new building wh. he is going to build, a plant for the freezing of bait so that the fishermen may go on catching fish after the natural run of the bait[61] is gone. Also the most successful of two Cooperative stores is here and the big schooner which the Cooperative Society own – the *Edward Blake* – is lying here and goes out this aft.

We have heard about the woman who came down to teach the knitting and weaving to the women. It is a total failure, the whole plan, and one, certainly, of the women this Miss Harris is conducting herself in a most absurd fashion. She writes notes to G. accusing him of being no gentleman because he does not advise attendance on her, as she deems fitting, meet her at wharves etc. And she has written saying that her trip is a great disappointment [to her. She expected] the course much more under his personal influence etc. She would be glad to take a cruise on the *Strathcona*, wd. not mind the hardships. etc. Imagine the situation. G. says it is the last of volunteer assistance for him in any capacity. It is enough to make one mad to see the inferiority of the service he gets out of anybody about him. It is partly his own fault. He is too erratic and bothers himself too little about detail. But this is the kind of people he gets.[62]

---

[61] The bait referred to is capelin, squid, herring, and mackerel.

[62] Grenfell had good service in this area from Jessie Luther who came to St. Anthony in 1906 and for the next four years was instrumental in setting up the Industrial Crafts section of the Grenfell Mission. As early as September 1906 crafts were ready for sale. Ms. Luther was followed in later years by Laura Young, Catherine Cleveland, Mae Alice Pressley-Smith, and others, including Anne Grenfell, who created an industry for the Grenfell Mission, which gave employment to many local women in northern Newfoundland and Labrador and was financially rewarding for the Mission (Paula Laverty, *Silk Stocking Mats: Hooked Mats of the Grenfell Mission*). In 1937, Grenfell wrote: "We have our own industrial school, and have 2000 workers in this one branch of our work…. We have shops in New York, Philadelphia and Boston and a tea-room at Middlebury, Vermont and at Cheshire, Connecticut which forms outlets for our handicrafts" (Joseph R.Smallwood, ed., *The Book of Newfoundland*. Vol. 1, p. 283).

This morning, the first thing that greeted G. was that two young Philadelphians, volunteers for his help, whom he had sent up Hare Bay to cut wood, had run his sloop aground up there and tramped home, and now, G. has got to go up there this afternoon and pull her off. And so it goes all the time. There is plenty of chance therefore for me to put a hand to this or that.

And yet he has ten times as much as he can do. He has 575 treatments on his book this season thus far, and he only began the 7th of June. It is twice as many as ever before, and will be far above a thousand before the end of September. It is the most interesting thing, to see when he steams into a harbor. It is not ten minutes till boats begin to come from every side. I counted 17 dories and punts made fast to our sides last night. You could not jump overboard without landing in one of them. He has little bights of rope, hanging every six or eight feet along his rail for them to catch hold of, and the men are aboard and have a painter about a stanchion before the anchor is down.

When you get into a bay it is quite impossible to say when you are going to get away. And this in part accounts for his singularly erratic way of arriving either before or after he said he would – generally, long after – never at the calculated time. Every man pays 25 cents, if he can. But many beg off and the receipts are small.

Your husband,
Edward C. Moore

WORKING AT ST. ANTHONY

S.S. *Strathcona*,
St. Anthony,
Sunday, July 30th.

My Dearest:

We made a day of it yesterday if ever. We were up at 5:00 and got 10 cords of wood on deck at Larks Cove in Hare Bay. The mosquitoes and flies were so bad we had to wear netting on our necks and put some kind of tar mixture on our hands. Then later in the day we had to get the same wood off the boat and pile it on the dock at St. Anthony. We steamed off to the little schooner which the party had last week when they came to grief. We got her off and towed her in to St. Anthony and beached her for repairs.

And finally, we got around from Goose Cove to the hospital, here a young man who is suffering from tuberculosis of the spine and is paralysed from the waist down and in the evening put a plaster jacket on him with the hope that some arrest may be secured in his disease. All this time the visits to the boats and the visiting on shore and the compounding of medicines etc. goes on almost without intermission. No men can be had for love or money to do the work which so much needs to be done here at St. Anthony. This will be the case so long as the fishing lasts. The chance of a haul wh. wd net $500.00 to a single boat in a single day – a thing which sometimes happens – possesses their imaginations and leads them to forget how many men have fished here a whole lifetime and never had a strike like that. But there is no use in talking about steady work and a dollar a day so long as the fishing is on.

And yet, if G. had twenty men here until the snow flies he could hardly do what he has planned. The wharf is unfinished, so is the orphanage, the fox run and bait freezer are not begun. The whole hot water plant for the hospital is not yet installed etc. If only a man with real head for affairs could stay here – and could get any helpers – the thing could be done.

The two young Philadelphia students are very willing. But not skilled at any of the trades involved, of course. The two women are at odds with one another, in a [bigway] that I would rather tell of than write of. It seems so infinitely foolish. Wrangling as to who is head of the house etc. It is very trying. And neither of them shows the slightest initiative to go ahead and get things in order. And tomorrow probably we go north and then, as G. despairingly says, nothing will be done until he comes back.

I preached at the little Methodist Ch. this morning and again this evening to a very good audience, and dined with G. at a Mr. John Moores house, the government customs inspector, and one of G's great helpers. I hold prayers on the ship every morning and every night, too, when the men can be got together. In the mornings it is all simple enough and everybody comes except the cook. We sing Moody and Sankey hymns and all the old favorites of the Portuguese Mission are coming back to me.

It is a nice set of fellows. But there are too many of us for so small a boat and too many different kinds of things go on, to make it easy to maintain any sort of order or cleanliness, and really, it is sometimes pretty trying.

G. had a beautiful salmon sent him today from a man to whose wife in her hour of need, as she lay in one corner of a one room house, with seven children already, on one fierce winter night a year ago, he gave his rug off his kometik as he chanced along in time to help her through.

From this place, Goose Cove nearby, he took up to Battle Harbor Hospital on his last trip, some years ago, before the hospital here was built, an elderly woman, very ill. She died under operation and he could not get word to her husband for several months. A year later, the man gave him $20.00 to bring back the body wh. had been buried in due form by a priest and in consecrated ground. Of course the body cannot be brought for a few years. But meantime in the consecrated ground in Goose Cove a stone sent up from St. Johns and bearing the inscription, – "Here lies the body" etc. wh. had been ordered at the same time with the order [given] G. to bring down the body.

A little boy helped us with the wood yesterday, aged fourteen years, the oldest of six and the only money getter for the whole household. His father died two years ago. His mother has 12.00 a year, aid from the govt. and she earned 12.00 at making seal-leather boots. That was all. I gave the boy a dollar, and I do not think I ever saw such happiness and gratitude in my life.

The little fellow, whose thigh was broken in an accident on a kometik three years ago, and of whom G. wrote the article, "Johnnie,"[63] in the magazine, brought to the boat yesterday a puppy for a present, the only thing in the world he could call his own.

Dearest love.

Yours,
E.C.M.

ST. ANTHONY TO BATTLE HARBOUR

Battle Harbor, Lab.
Tuesday evening, Aug.1st.

My Dearest Wife:

I wrote you on Sunday from St. Anthony. But it seemed best to bring all the letters here and let them go back by the next *Home* on Saturday. There is no mail from St. Anthony for 10 days.

---

[63] The magazine referred to could have been *Among the Deep Sea Fishers*, a periodical of the Grenfell Mission's activities, which was set up in 1903 in support of Grenfell's work. It ceased publication in 1981. It could also have been the magazine *Toilers of the Deep*, which included early Grenfell writings.

The two patients there were getting on finely. The man in the plaster jacket had more relief than he has known for a year and had some signs of recovery of partial use of his legs. It came out on Sunday that he had been to the hospital in St. Johns and been refused. At least it was so reported. When he was questioned it came out that though that was not true, he had made the long journey to a place near St. Johns, in order to let his spine be rubbed by the hands of a man who was the seventh consecutive son of his mother. Such seventh sons, if only the line have been not been broken by a daughter, are reputed to be healers, and to work cures of all sorts by magic or miracle. They are not allowed to receive compensation, of course, but there is no way of preventing their receiving presents. I tried to find out if it was an Indian superstition. But the figure seven indicates rather that it is of Christian origin, probably an English old-wives fable.

The other case was that of a man with a fearfully swelled and discolored arm, septic to his shoulder, probably from a wound in the hand when splitting fish – the water around the stages becomes so incredibly foul, and the mens blood is often so impoverished. This man came from Red Bay on the Labrador side of the Straits. In a day or two he wd. have lost his arm and before long his life. Six men brought him over in a row-boat sixty five miles, and then quietly rowed back. They would be gone from their fishing three days, at the time of year when if they do not catch fish they will be poor to the point of starvation for a whole year. The season is so very short, and this is just the height of it. And yet they did not seem to think they were doing anything great.

In the same manner, this evening, as we were steaming along through the dense fog and thinking we must be getting somewhere near the opening for Battle Harbor, we suddenly met a trap-skiff – bigger than the biggest whale boat you ever saw – with four men rowing, and soon discovered that the man who was steering was Dr. Simpson. He was on his way to Henley Harbor – or, as everybody here says – "'Enley 'Arbor", – to see a man who from the descriptions he surmised had typhoid fever. Typhoid is very common here because the people are so incredibly careless about the water supply, and drainage etc.

Well, here were these five men in the welter of a huge Labrador sea. Dense fog, ice bergs all around, rocks, reefs everywhere, in an open boat. They had come twenty-eight miles to get S. would row him down and then tomorrow bring him back and then return themselves, 112 miles to row. Of course they have their little bark-tanned jigger sails. But there was no wind all day yesterday. Only this terrific wallow of a sea from the end of the world and nothing visible five rods ahead of you for hours together, never a buoy, fog-horn, whistle, spile,[64] not to say light house, for a hundred miles at a stretch. We turned back and gave them ten miles of a tow line, and so set them on their way. Whereat they were grateful, you may be sure.

Simpson and the skipper came aboard, and we had a good talk with them. But thereby we were two hours late in getting to the Southern Tickle here and had our own time in the fog and almost pitchy darkness getting in. But of that later. The Governor was at Henley and Grenfell urged Simpson to go to him, tell him the whole story, get him to see the case – he happens to be a doctor himself. And perhaps he will send Simpson back on the *Faiona*, the government yacht in wh. he is travelling.

Sunday we went to see the little boy – one of eleven children – of Grenfells old komatik man named Simms, a great trapper and woodsman, but a man who has never had any luck with fishing. But this man has this year taken – along with two share-men – nearly five hundred quintals of fish. All last week they took them so fast that they could not dress between night and morning what they took between morning and night. They were almost completely exhausted at the end of the week.

---

[64] A spile can be a wooden stake. In this context, it may mean a place where a ship could have safe anchorage.

And Saturday night they let go from the trap what he estimated at twenty five quintals – because next day was Sunday and they would not keep till Monday without the first dressing[65] and not a fish is ever dressed on Sunday. It was to him like a law of nature. But I wonder if it would have been so in Gloucester, or anywhere among our fishermen with such a chance to make what was to him a fortune and only the Sunday sentiment to prevent. Just on that part of the shore many other men have done nearly as well and the season is one of great prosperity. On the southern side of Newfoundland and on the west side of the Straits, on the other hand the run has been poor.

It is curious that nothing has any value, except cod. Fresh salmon are sold for 25 cts a piece – weighing sometimes 25 to 40 pounds – Cured salmon brings only 2 cts a pound. Lobsters are a cent a piece – and the natives never eat them, and salmon they serve rather under protest to their visitors, but dont care much for themselves. Ducks are rank and fishy – but it is not the season yet of course.

A miserable, scrawny lamb was killed for the boat the other day and deemed a great luxury. But you can see by what I have said that the living on the boat has not been half as bad as it was represented. Only that one does miss vegetables and fruit – just a little once in a great while – and eggs are unknown. Nothing is so bad about the boat as the dirt. She is filthy – I cannot say less – She can hardly be less so long as she is a menagerie – and G. is so devoted to his pets. He is going to keep the foxes on board until the end of the season.

She carries everything, fire-wood, coal, lumber, all on her decks, beside freight of every description. And the crew is too small for what is expected of them. And G. is more erratic and…disorderly than any man I ever knew. He does not care in the least for any thinkable form of discomfort. And I like that. I can stand that, too. But I never saw an Englishman who was so indifferent to dirt.

And rarely have I seen a man who had less capacity for delegating

---

[65] Gut out and head off.

work. Choosing good subordinates or giving them any kind of chance and responsibility when he had chosen them. He thinks he has given instructions when he has never opened his hand. Never explains his plans, and then is surprised because things do not get forward in his absence but is certain to bring up standing anybody who does go ahead. He carries far more work than he can long endure and cannot seem to delegate any of it. This is the rock on which the whole large venture is going to split if he does not develop other qualities than he thus far has shown.

At St. Anthony, everything is at sixes and sevens. The crew of the Co-operator mutinied and he had to put on board of her the three men whom he had engaged for the season, three carpenters etc. And he has nobody there now except a slow, old man as general trusty, the two college students – Penn. Univ. – and the two women. Which latter two are at swords points with one another, hardly speaking except to quarrel. Miss H. who is housekeeper refusing to let the servants take orders from Miss K. who is the head nurse. So that hospital slops stand on the steps all day, just where Miss H. told the maid to put them down etc. etc. And outside – what with dock, orphanage, fox-run drainage, etc. there is work for 20 men under a competent all-round supt. until the snow flies.

I cleaned up the store house, opened some sixty cases – failed, to find Kingman's lost cases by the way – made memoranda of contents of many which I half nailed up again. Sent many things up to house and hospital and some things aboard. What with this and the handling of cord wood and the getting off the ledge of the stranded schooner, known as the *Arts*, my hands are a good deal like what they were when I came home from Whitemarshs cruise.

It will some day be a great plant at St. Anthony – and the saw-mill, wh. we did not see – and which is only 25 miles away, should be counted with it. He has contracts for 300,000 feet of sawed lumber if he can get it out. But he has almost no men there now. They will not work when they can fish – and when they do not fish they are used to a very desultory lazy life – But it is all far from being a great plant yet, and it never will be until it has real superintendence.

I was glad enough to be told we were to sail at 4:30 a.m. Tuesday – with two poor wrecks of women in the ship, hospital. G. was low in his mind at having failed to see the governor – no royal governor has ever in history visited this end of the island – and this one had promised.

At 5:30 we met the *Faiona* with the Governor aboard going in to St. Anthony. Grenfell put about, landed at once – so did the Gov. – took him on a tour of inspection of every blessed thing, hospital, house, library, dispensary, laundry, school, not a living soul except the poor servants out of bed – imagine the feelings of the American ladies, who were ever so disappointed at not having had the amount of attention they expected – governors arriving while they were in bed.

Grenfell, who had been so cavalier and scrubby, all pleasure and grace – four or five drawling young Englishmen at his heels, – "Well, I say, now, by jove, rather fine, this, old boy," etc. fifty Esquimaux dogs at their heels, packing boxes everywhere, looms half set up, in the parlor, reed-organ taken to pieces by one of the Penn. boys and not yet got together again…was on the stairs, gut I presume it was. Coal all over our decks just as the men knocked off the night before, one of the little foxes washed through a hawse-hole in the two inch stream from the hose wherewith we were trying to trim the ship while the gov. visited the ladies – cooks boy put off to get him.

Gov. came aboard – still only about 7:30 o'clock – rather keen looking old Scot – Sir William McGregor – not a bed made yet, of course. But the skipper had thought that the damp in the cabin shd. be relieved, ordered a little fire in the vile little stove wh. until hot never does anything but smoke. G. very much vexed at that, goes off to *Faiona* to breakfast with Sir William.

Comes back radiant. Gov. truly interested in everything. Will get grant for drainage of whole St. Anthony plant – much needed – and pretty surely grant for a new Hospital at Harrington, a scheme he had much at the [heart of his plans]. And – what is most to our purpose – he has accomplished his conference with his Excellency so that we do not have to go and hang about Chateau, but are able to head straight for Battle.

Should have been in long before dark but for giving the tow to Simpson. As it was arrived about 8:45 beginning to be dark. Dense fog, heavy sea – arrived off, I mean, emerged from, fog – to feel the land – about a mile too far south, had the greatest difficulty to make out where we were and keep off rocks while doing it, passed between two enormous ice bergs both stranded and one breaking up in the pounding sea, found the mouth of the tickle and went in through a channel not 30 feet wide in places.

Croucher, the agent on the wharf, said not a man lived on the coast wd do that after dark except Grenfell. But the alternative was bad – to anchor very difficult, water far too deep so soon as you are off shore a bit, and to cruise up and down, measuring with the log all night, otherwise feasible, but very dangerous now because of all this ice.

Stumbled upon G. at the house and found your letters of the 16th and 19th-20th and mothers of 23rd and your telegram of 24th…. Oh, what a joy and what a relief it was. And dear Dorothea's letter so sweet. I have read every one of them all many times.

I slept in a bed at the hospital – my bunk was becoming intolerable. – It is now Wed. aft. that I am writing.

There are four cases here to be operated on including the two we brought. So we shall not get away until Friday morning, that is certain. But then we expect to go to Indian Harbor for Sunday. There the gov. overtakes us and he wants to push on with a fast cruise to Cape Chidley, if the ice will permit.

You see how it is. No one can tell when anything will take place. Even the eclipse may not take place on time up here – and that is my only hope of getting back before Christmas, that G. has promised by all that is holy to help the Lick[66] Observatory people at Sandwich Bay with their observation of the eclipse. But if air and exercise are what I came for, I am getting these. Am well beyond belief and really deeply interested in what I see. So relieved to hear of you and all you are doing. [I received] mothers letter today with yours of 20th – by way of St. Johns. Send always to Battle.

Dearest, loving,
Edward C. Moore

OF BOYS AND DOGS

Battle Harbor, Labrador,
August 2nd.

My Dear Little Boy:

My letters from home, which I received when we got here last night, brought me very near to you all, and made me feel what I was missing in not being with you at Punkey. It was all so lovely then and we were so happy there. Perhaps some other summer we may go back there. Mother says you had a nice visit from Will and then grandmas visit must have been a great pleasure, and then I understand that Grandpa Brown came and took you all to Rockland and I suppose he was taking you on that wonderful journey on his railroad. And then Dorothea went to Newhark and you and mother to Seal Harbor, and then Pasque and finally Orange and there I hope to come and find you. What a summer you have had, my dear boy, so much that was beautiful and happy in it. Few little guys, you know, have as much.

---

66   The Lick Observatory is located on Mount Hamilton in California. It is part of the University of California and primarily a research institution. It was founded in 1888 through the legacy of the California millionaire, James Lick. Some of its people were sent to Cartwright to observe the solar eclipse in 1905 (http://mthamilton.ucolick.org).

But ever since I reached this coast I have been wishing that some day I might bring you here, just as I want some day to bring you to the beautiful mountains in Switzerland which I love so dearly. And strangely enough though here I am always on the sea, there is much in the place which reminds me of Switzerland, always rocks and ice and snow – and many things in the houses and in the lives of the people remind me of Switzerland.

Do you remember that last year, when you sent your dollar up here, a Doctor Simpson sent you a lovely little letter in reply. Well, he is sitting opposite to me now and wishes to be remembered to you. And Mrs. Simpson sends you these photographs of the dear little boy who was almost eaten up by the dogs. These were taken when he was in the Hospital at Indian Harbor and the lady is Mrs. Simpson. He was the agent's son – agent of the Hudson Bay Fur-Trading Company – at their Post at Cartwright, about eighty miles from Indian Harbor.

It was winter and the dogs were very savage – they look just like great wolves – and, though the people could never get through a winter here without them nobody ever trusts them. Well, perhaps you heard Dr. Grenfell tell the story at our house last winter. The little boy was standing with his father near the store-house of the Post and the father was talking to an Indian and without a moments warning one big dog jumped on the little boy, and the moment he was down on the ground all the dogs were on him biting and tearing.

The father would not even take a second to get a club but fought the pack with his fists and boots, and the Indian clubbed them with his gun and when he had broken that in pieces he stabbed them right and left with his hunting knife. The father was dressed in skins and so escaped bad bites but once they had him on the ground. And though it was all over in a minute, when they carried the little boy in, he had thirty-seven different bites. They did what they could for him. But when they found he was not getting better, they hitched up a komatik with ten dogs – not the same ones – and drove those eighty miles to the Hospital. The dogs which had attacked him, they shot every one of them – for they felt they could never trust them again.

Somewhere up here two men were travelling together each with a loaded komatik and his own train of dogs, and the one thought he would go over and ride with the other on the komatick so they could talk together. He thought he could drive his own with his long lash. As he jumped off his sledge, he stumbled and fell in the deep snow. And before he could get up his own dogs were all over him. The other team got excited and joined in the fray, and it was all the two men could do to save themselves.

They make the strangest noises you ever heard when they howl, especially at night. And when one begins they all join, and you would think the whole town was being invaded by wolves. And yet you see, there are no roads – not a foot of road in this whole part of the world. In summer one goes everywhere in a boat, or if it is inland one has to cut his way through forest or wade up the valley of streams. But in winter the streams are all frozen solid for six or seven months and deep snow with hard crust covers everything except the higher trees in the forest, and even the sea has a rim of shore ice which is often safe to travel. Men venture across bays as much as ten or even twenty miles wide all frozen over. Then a man with a sledge and train of dogs can go anywhere.

Thus they do almost all their travelling, then they drag down logs from the forest and move stores and building material – and all by the aid of dogs. Not a horse lives on all this coast. He never could travel the snow. There would be nothing he could eat the most of the year, and the dogs would kill him in a moment if they caught him alone. Mother will read you parts of my journal to her. But I wanted you to have a little letter of your own and to know how I love you and how I long to see you and how happy I am in all that mother says about your being such a dear good boy, so courteous and gentlemanly, so obedient and kind. Ah, my dear boy, I pray for you night and morning that God will bless you and keep you and make a great and good man of you in His service.

With dearest love. Your father.
Edward C. Moore.

A LOVE LETTER

Battle Harbor,
August 3rd.

My Darling:

We are off before noon. Everything has been rushed through at top speed. Grenfell is in such a fever now that he has lost so much time. And the Governor follows in the *Faiona* in a day or two and is anxious to get as far as Cape Chidley, the entrance to Hudsons Bay. And G. will seek to do most of his visiting on the way back. So we are cutting ourselves off almost as much as if we were going into the wilderness. And no one knows how we are going to get back from Cartwright or Indian Harbor to Battle to catch the *Home*.

But, if this plan gets us to Domino on the way back, as it well may we shall take the *Virginia Lake* there on the 23rd and get the *Home* here on the 26th. Which is a week earlier than I said before. If not, we shall have to come [to Cartwright and] take our chances on an excursion boat, after the eclipse. I am sure we shall manage it somehow though no one can tell us just how. The Hudson Bay Co's. agent at Cartwright will know all about ships at the last moment.

But I cannot let this mail go without thanking you unspeakably for every line in your dear letters. I have read every one of them three or four times over. And your letters tell me you were all safe so far as the 24th and lets me know all your plans. I only think as I read what a load of care and responsibility I have left you with while I am here in this irresponsible way. Oh Bessie dear it is not right willing as you are to take it and infinitely readily and well as you do most things. You had such a year, last year and you have had no rest and…summer has been made to [lend] to this Labrador plan for me. I have a sort of second sense about it therefore as a thing which I must do to my very best because it is costing you so much. But it is not right.

I could see your every move at dear old Punkey, and I am so grateful to you for mother's visit, and Frank's, and for your aid through

Metcalf to Charles. You will let me pay half of that, will you not? It is a great thing when I think how you made your way to Yonkers and then to Providence and then to Diannes place, and I think that they must think so too. And then comes the closing up at Punkey with all the details, for some of which at least I could help you. Then, Seal Harbor for you and Hans and Newhark for Dorothea and meantime, Rockland and, I suppose, the Aroostook trip, for one or both of them and then Pasque and then Orange.

I can hardly bear not to be with you a day at Pasque. But it will be good to be beside you in Orange, where we began. And If you want to perhaps we can go off somewhere for a few days. But, all the time, there is the Kirkland St. house to think of and plan for…. I cannot tell you how…to go off thus so far and so long and leave you and everything.

I cannot tell you how I long for you, turn to you, think of you and of the future and recall the past and always it is your figure and your fun which is the light and glory of it all. I do think as you say that we have come to a great…lives and I cannot say how I long and pray to make you happy and give you praise and blessing in the years before us. It is much that has been given to us and we must get the good out of it as it goes.

Here, Mr. Moore refers to the hopes of their relationship which are faith-related and to their attempt to live Christian ideals in helping others and in raising their children together. He philosophizes on the pitfalls on the road of life and he continues:

When that is the case one does not do for others all that one might or exert on them just the influence one would. It is a great chance we now have for ourselves and for our children, and I long to enter into it with you. I bless you for every word you say about the dear children as being so good and sweet and helpful. My arms around you. Do you miss me as I miss you? Tenderest love and deepest prayer.

Your Husband,

E.

PROCURING SOME FURS

Battle Harbor,
August 3rd, Thurs.

My Darling:

There is just a bare chance that an answer to this may meet me at
Battle on my way back – directed here of course. It is just a chance of
course, and of no great consequence. I have been looking at a great
choice of skins wh. Simpson has. And have picked out 2 lynx skins,
at $7.00 each, and a red fox at 7.00 and a gray fox – patch – at 20.00.
The last wd. be worth 200.00 if it were all silver as 9/10 of it is, i.e.
if it had not a rusty place or two on neck and belly – just a touch
of tawny hair. But it was an enormous fox, with a wonderful brush.
Altogether, it is a very fine skin. That makes $41.00, they come in
duty free and the mounting as rugs etc. does not cost – Kingman
thinks he recalls his own – more than 2.50 or 3.00 each.

I am leaving the skins here and am not paying until I come back lest
I should see something elsewhere. But what I particularly want to
know is if you want an otter – like the collar of my fur coat – very
beautiful skin $20.00. I do not know if ladies are using them for
collars or anything of that sort. If so, I shd. like to give you one.
And perhaps one for May though I thought of giving her one of the
lynxs for her floor. The otter skins are about 3 ft long and nearly
two ft wide best in the middle of course but very handsome. Too
handsome for anything but furs to wear. But if you or M or Dorothea
can wear them I will get one or two. If I do not hear from you that
you think them available for wearing I will not buy them, for of
course, we can always send to Simpson or Grenfell. In great haste,
just as we go. And with tenderest love, and hurrying, longing for you
all the time.

Your husband,
Edward.

ALONG THE COAST OF LABRADOR

S.S. *Strathcona*,
Off Batteau, Lab.
Sat. Aug. 5th.

My Dear Wife:

I wrote you in what was supposed to be our last moment at Battle Harbor. But just then a schooner came in wh. had some coal – we were short – so we stayed the afternoon for coaling, and then slept aboard so as to be able to start at dawn on Friday. – I had been sleeping at the Hospital those two nights that we were there. The beds on the ship are something terrible – Mine is a frame of gas pipe six feet long by eighteen inches wide hung by ropes from the deck frame and covered with sail cloth bent on with cord through the eyelets. Kingmans is eighteen inches above mine.

I learned that Simpson had a funeral that afternoon and I offered to take it as there was an operation at once ordered which he wanted to see. It was the funeral of a little boy, two months old, fourth child and first son of a young couple – this other woman looked to be 45. I hear she is 27. The child had died rather suddenly. The father was away on the other shore fishing and did not get word for a day or two.

The house was of the very poorest. But the plain little box for a coffin was covered with white muslin and trimmed with black braid and there was a wreath of paper flowers wh. Simpson says belongs to the woman in the place who aids on all such occasions and the wreath appears at every funeral. Two small boys had white scarves around their caps and acted as bearers, feeling their importance very much. I read the English service at their request and made a prayer when I learned that the mother was not to go to the grave.

After that we walked down through the fish house – even on such occasions not to be escaped with its terrible odor and its slippery floor – got into a trap-skiff – in the same condition as the stage – the father and two of his friends rowed. A grandmother and half a dozen children went with us. We were rowed out round the reef, landed on the next island, walked across the incredibly barren rocks and the soggy peat in their crevices to the little grave yard with its high stockade to keep out the dogs.

There is no soil in this part of the world. And when you dig down a few inches into the peat the water drains into your excavation from the rocks on every side. You have to dig in the hollows, or there would be no peat. This little grave, so pathetically small, was full of water when we arrived, had to be bailed out while we stood, and was practically full again before we left. In other words, even when people die on land up here they do not escape being buried in water. I do not [know] when I have done anything which moved me more.

One thing impresses me with the people in all their relations. They are so used to contending against a world wh. is so much too strong for them, where all the forces are so fierce and wild and cruel and overwhelming, they are so used not to having their own way or setting their own wills through that, hardy as they are, there is a kind of blank submissiveness about them, too. It is so noticeable in the way in wh. they meet their poverty and in the way in wh. they meet sickness and death. I have not seen as much writhing or heard as much groaning, as most people we know do at a toothache. And hardly have seen a tear – but such faces of patient, silent woe.

We got away at 3:30 next morning – it is broad daylight at that hour here – had a heavy, heavy sea and no end of ice, fifty bergs in sight at a given moment – many aground and going to pieces. It is this shore ice which has played such havoc with what otherwise wd. have been a good season for most. Hugh chunks, or the bergs themselves, float down resistlessly into the traps and nets, tear them to pieces or force the fishers to rush out and take them up, just after they have put them down.

And the other day at Francis Harbor three men, a father and two sons, were trying to save their trap – their only capital – from a big berg, when a piece fell off it into their boat, smashed the boat to match sticks and killed them all.

At Square Islands we went ashore and while the Dr. visited sick, I went up to the school where a young college student, a Methodist from St. Johns, was holding school two months in the summer. He has 22 children from the village, but only 11 were present – older ones help on stages when there is any pressure. Women work everywhere on the stages up here with a skirt of old oilers over their dresses. You can imagine the filth and the exposure of the women. One side of the shack where the school was was against the hill and the other sides were poles covered with sods. It had only paper windows, being used only in summer, and was as wet as everything else.

I talked with the young man, a Newfoundlander by birth. Only reading and writing and a little arithmetic to teach of course. But the schools are supported by the Methodist Conference and have a subvention from the government at places where the government has no schools. With such opportunities to learn in their youth, you wonder at the demand for reading matter, which the Mission meets.

Hardly a man ever comes on deck who does not ask for papers, magazines and books. And Grenfell puts down and takes up little libraries of twenty to fifty volumes – all kinds of books – in a box with a list and which stay in a place for a winter and are moved on to some other place next winter. I have been arranging some of these and making lists etc. as we have cruised. But we shall distribute forty or fifty boxes of magazines, reviews etc. besides wh. the people keep – and often paper their houses with the pictures, just as I have seen nurseries papered, or like a picture screen.

If G's secretary was of any use whatever this part of the work would all be done automatically, for nothing cd. be simpler. But always there is friction about it, and a deadly aversion on the part of the youth to any literature but tracts. Grenfell has a circular concerning consumption, forbidding spitting etc. – a universal vice – even the women spit like lobsters – wh. circular he has ordered to go with every handful of literature. But it is always being forgotten and left out.

I went later to visit a woman who is dying of pneumonia, far gone but entirely conscious. Mother of five young children, father with her, a nice old man, husband not much good, G. said. She seemed so grateful to have me read and pray with her. Such a hovel, and not a breath of air in her room, perfectly stifling.

G. bought five more foxes for his fox farm. But fortunately brought only one of the new ones aboard. Got in to Venison Tickle for the night, passed a huge ice berg aground at the entrance and a small one lay in the middle of the narrow roadstead, near where we must anchor. Very rotten it was, all mushroom formed from having been eaten away by the sea, must have been carried in by the tide, but seemed to be aground.

Went ashore after we anchored to see the old agent and the big stores. Halket, the agent, has been here forty years and is something of a character all up and down the coast. While we were there it began to rain and was pitchy dark. Just as we were on the dock and climbing down into the boat, there was a tremendous crash and a large part of the mushroom toppled over. We waited for the commotion to subside and pushed off in the boat and as we passed the berg it seemed to us that it was moving. Sure enough, the diminution of weight and change in the centre of gravity had set it afloat, and the tide was bearing it.

We got aboard and ordered steam up, so that we might move our berth if necessary though the place was so narrow that it seemed difficult to see where we should go. We watched the uncanny white thing for a long time and then concluded to go below, leaving one man to watch. But nobody wanted to get into bed. It seemed too likely that we should have to get out in a hurry. Sure enough, after a half an hour, and just as one of us was going up the ladder to have a last look, the man came running to the companion-way, saying, "She is coming down on us, sir."

We got up anchor and before the anchor was in the chains, the thing seemed as if it wd. touch the bowsprit. We had begun to move astern, and when under way drew off to the other side of the channel and got out a stern line to a schooner there to prevent our stern from swinging out against the iceberg. Two men were put to watch. And this morning before breakfast another huge piece fell off. It will all break up today I should think. But it was too close quarters to be comfortable.

Here at Seal Islands we fell in with a young fellow, a Harvard graduate of the last class, Webster, who has charge of the kerosene launch wh. the N.Y. men gave Grenfell last winter[67] and is now leased to the Marconi people while they are getting their line in order. He seemed a very fine fellow. But he had had no end of trouble with his crew, two Battle Harbor men who were sick of their contract, and I honestly think were afraid to put to sea in the thing after one or two experiences which they had had. She seemed so tiny for such work. I did not blame them much for kicking at the constant wet and discomfort. But I think they were afraid, too.

This is Sunday afternoon at Batteau. There are seventy five craft in the harbor and if one reckons ten people to the schooner, as is fair, it makes quite a population. But yet only three families are 'liveyers', that is remain here the year round. And they are of half Esquimaux blood and the…people we have seen. The people from the schooners live mostly in sod-huts made of poles and stones, and the sick among them have a hard time.

The two doctors are off now on an operation for a poor man, who can hardly live, and whose brother has been kept from fishing the whole time that they have been here by nursing him. There will be a woman with a tumor to take on to Battle Harbor when we go tomorrow. I visited this morning a woman whose baby had died

---

[67] Many small launches were donated to Grenfell to serve on the Labrador coast. The first of these was the *Princess Mary* which was donated in 1893. Later, a bigger ship, the *Maraval*, was donated to the International Grenfell Association by a lady in New York and served the Labrador coast for many years. Dr. Paddon had the use of this vessel to serve his district around North West River and Indian Harbour (Wilfred Grenfell, *A Labrador Doctor*, pp. 267 & 288).

a few weeks ago. The little body is preserved in salt in the fish house, to be taken back to Newfoundland after the season is over. She herself is in wretched condition.

The catch has been good here. But the number of sore wrists which I have seen goes ahead of anything you can imagine and the filth of this little harbor with all these people cleaning their fish into it, scores of tons of fish every day for six weeks, can better be imagined than described.

I conducted the service this morning and shall again this evening. I went this afternoon, to a praise and experience meeting, the most pronounced 'Methody'[68] I have ever seen. As pronounced as any I have ever seen among the negroes at the south. I was a good deal surprised for these are all Newfoundland people and all English. It was rather pitiful in a way. But after all the main thing is that it does keep up the moral tone of their lives in conditions which sadly test that tone.

Almost all the boats bring down girls to cook and split fish because men are so hard to get for any work at this time of the year, and women's work is so much cheaper. But whether on board or in the sod-huts on shore the conditions are sadly dangerous for them and the misery among them is awful.

We got started on a discussion at breakfast this morning which brought out Grenfells Moodyish side more than I ever saw it, and… of course in any [discussion] he only sees one side of the question. But it is sad that he shd. be so intolerant. I must keep off that subject – and a few others – in future. It is the old-fashioned Church of England Evangelical, with all his limitations and all of his splendid qualities.

As I try to fit into a plan on the ship and in her work, I also come into collision with the quality wh makes it so hard for others to work with him – viz. that you never can tell what he is going to do next – for the most excellent will in the world [is unable to know]. He

---

[68] Slang reference to the evangelistic, Methodist movement of Charles and John Wesley and George Whitfield.

does not know himself. And he cannot delegate work in the least or live with the slightest expectation that anybody will carry anything out. So that the result is that while he is running round, knocked from one imperative decision to another in a way that wears him pitifully, the people who should help him and also those who gladly would help him, stand by idly because they have not the slightest idea what he wants or what he needs. And are likely to be blamed for not divining something that is beyond any human divination.

His skipper is a most admirable all round man but he is going to lose him because one moment he treats him like a cabin boy, and the next goes off and forgets everything, and when he comes back rakes him roundly for not having taken all the responsibilities and [forecast] of the master of the ship. And so it goes in everything.

I am trying to remember some of the funny stories of patients which I hear.

A tuberculous patient, being told, the other day, that he must be fed up, said, "But not with them nutriments, Doctor, I wants a hunk of fat 'swile' – seal – or a fish-gull. Now, that would have some taste."

The man of all work at Battle came to Kingman the other day and [asked], "Doctor, can you shove some tow into the seams of my teeth?"

The English has certain very marked peculiarities e.g. the use of the pronouns in the nominative when they should be in the accusative, "I pays he for he's trap."

And of the little foxes the cabin boy said to me the other day – "He fit, – fought – he wonderful."

A man brought on board last night the largest polar bear skin I ever saw. The bear was shot within five miles of here last winter. Came down on an ice floe, and when the ice broke up, swam ashore, and started north again on the rocks. "He were heading straight home, he were, when I shot he." Unfortunately, he wants a price as big as the pelt, and it is not particularly well cured and the claws are gone.

I am going to mail this here tomorrow morning before we leave for I cannot send again for almost two weeks. It seems a very long time until the end of August. But I do not want to make you unhappy. It is a pretty rough life – I do not mind that – But it is such close quarters – for grown men to be thrown into for so long a time. I do not think boys mind that so much. But I think I do. And it is so incredibly dirty and every conceivable thing so needlessly so. Of course G. has his mind on other things, so he ought to have. But his captain would do all this, if G. really wanted him [to].

I am wonderfully well, eating and sleeping perfectly. Sometimes getting very hard exercise, sometimes, suffering for want of it. But you must think of me as just as well as possibly can be and doing everything and waiting for everything for your dear sake. But, oh, so unspeakably glad when I can get away and start back. I hope my letters prove a little what you would like to know. If not I think they must be insufferable bore, they are so long.

Dearest, your husband,
ECM.

EXPERIENCING THE ISOLATION OF THE COAST

Nearing Indian Harbor,
Tuesday, Aug. 8th.

My Dearest:

I left a letter for you at Batteau to go up by the *Virginia Lake*. But we learn that she has not yet passed Indian Harbor. So that I will have this ready to go with her if we catch her. She is the last mail boat until the one which carries us away after the eclipse. Her arrival should be two weeks. But it will be prolonged to then in order to get the eclipse parties away. At least so we are told. And…the alternative is to get Miss Edgar's excursion ship, the *Practrona*, which witnesses the eclipse in Cartwright, when we go. Also to take us to Battle and there we get the *Home*. In either case I must keep my journal now to bring with me as, if I send it, it will not get there until after I do. And yet it is a month today until the very earliest that I can hope to see you.

And it gave me a strange feeling last night as we passed the Marconi pole at Domino that that was the last possibility of communication with you either to or fro, until we come out again more than three weeks hence. Oh I hope things go well with you. We sent a boat in to inquire, but they had no messages for us.

I told you about our Sunday at Batteau. Grenfell saw almost a hundred cases from Sat. evg. until early Monday morning. The fishermen have had a splendid season, most of them, and are very happy. One crew of eight men, lying near us, had fourteen-hundred quintals of fish and last year they brought $3.70 to the fishermen himself per quintal.

The two hospital patients came aboard early. One poor Irish woman with a tumor, and a man with a chronic appendical trouble. Then we got away.

At Spotted Islands we were met in the channel by a man who wanted G. to see his son – the last of nine sons – the next last was drowned last fall while gunning. At Domino we were picked up in the same way by a boat containing a young man who had the worst ulcer from a molar tooth I have ever seen. It was just breaking to discharge through his cheek.

At Domino the *Faiona* with the Governor aboard caught up with us. We went on to Gready where G. expected some sick and when we came up from breakfast, the *Faiona* was steaming in. As result of consultation, G. went aboard of her and will go with her to Cartwright and we are on the way to Indian Harbor direct. We shall make about eighty miles today. The *Faiona* can go so much faster than we that this was an economy of time. And we are already so disappointingly late. We shall not get further down the coast than to Nain, the Moravian Mission to the Esquimaux, even if we get so far. G. never has any plan or books aboard, and his going with the governor introduces an element very difficult to calculate.

It is the first bright day we have had since the first Sunday at Battle – no fog anywhere – less ice than we had seen to the south, and a warmer air, less wintry and biting than anything I have felt since I left Sydney. There has been through the latter part of the afternoon a wonderful mirage making the island and the shore look very strange.

"Now," says the sailor on the watch, "now, sir, the h'island is coming out like he's self again. It is the h'air sir – the h'atmosphere. It do do wonderful tings 'ere."

Said a man last night of a patient – "I reckon he do be fair bad, by now."

Said an old man Sunday when I had seated myself in the stern – he wished to scull – "I don't know how I can propagate the boat, sir."

"It is fair good money for the likes of we," says a fisherman of his expectation of turning his fish to cash in St. Johns.

"h'ice-h'islands" is the regular name of ice bergs.

The contrary of "forward" is "h'aft" always.

The habit of saying "They be," "he be" leads them to say "he be's long" for he belongs.

G. was examining the sputum last night of a boy of 14 whom he had visited Sunday on his father's boat in Batteau Harbor. The boy is far gone in consumption. Before they came away, two months ago, they sent for a Doctor near their Newfoundland home. He said in a rather tried, but at bottom friendly manner, "Why d – n, it all, why did not you send for me earlier. You d – n, procrastinating, stingy people wait and wait and now, d – n me if I think I can save your boy."

The boy was so deeply offended at the profanity that he flatly refused to take any of the Doctor's medicine, and they had to send for another from 40 miles distant, at $50.00 cost – who could only tell them the same thing in less profane way.

But it was the religious feeling of the boy about the swearing wh. determined his attitude. It is a marvel to me how deeply religious those are who are religious at all, how outwardly respectful all are, although of course there are many reckless and tough characters among them and certain vices show themselves in horrid ways among them. But drunkenness is not one of these. There is almost no liquor to get. And even the bad Englishman is not so bad as when he is in liquor as at home.

I am afraid there is never going to be any time for going ashore for fishing, hunting or tramping. There is such a pressure of the medical work and whenever it slacks off – it is up anchor and away to the next place. So that any longer expeditions are impossible. But I do want to see a little bit of the interior of this land of which we shall have seen so many hundred miles of this iron-bound, forbidding and mysterious coast.

If I bring back my mint rod and net, without ever having unpacked them, I can exchange them for an axe for Hans and some other things of the kind. I want to get a black bear skin for you if I can, and a white seal. I shall surely have a chance. Grenfell took the half breed's polar bear skin at 70.00 and he expects to dispose of it to some of the eclipse people for 100.00. It would bring 200.00 in America. It is perfectly enormous – as is also the smell of it, as it occupies a store room next our bunks and the partition does not reach to the ceiling.

My blue flannel suit, the old one is about used up and the knickerbockers beginning to show the wear. The rest I shall bring back with me of course. I should have felt somewhat differently about the trip except that G. has gone to Cartwright. He expected to be in wireless communication all the time. But with the breakdown between Chateau and Battle that has proven impossible of course. And so here we are steaming away from you as fast as we can for three whole weeks and more beyond all reach. I shall be glad when it is over. I do not think we can fail of one or the other of the connections I spoke of, and that means arriving on the morning of the 8th of Sept. – your birthday.

But if the sailing day of the *Home* shd. be changed – or any one of a half-dozen other things happen – we might be delayed. I will telegraph you – to Orange? I suppose – just so soon as I am in wire communication, Chateau – Bay of Islands or North Sydney. This last wd. mean that I [will arrive] by rail from Boston. Oh, how glad I shall be. I feel as if in this letter I am taking a last farewell of you. For after this no letters will go from this coast – and perhaps not even this. Hug my children for me. And believe, believe my darling wife, in my great love for you.

Your husband,
Edward C. Moore.

LONELINESS AND LONGING

Strathcona,
Indian Harbor, Lab.
August 8th.

My Darling:

Here we are at anchor and have taken the two patients ashore – the woman in a pitiable condition – and made all preparations that can be made for tomorrow. And we have found that the *Virginia Lake*, the mail boat, has not been here. In fact, we have caught up with Wood, the London secretary of the M.D.S.F.[69] and he is going south on the *V.L.*[70] So you see I can send another letter. It is pretty clear that the *V.L.* has got through this time to Nain, the

---

[69] Mission to Deep Sea Fishermen

[70] *Virginia Lake*

Moravian Mission to the Esquimaux wh. is her last point of call and which she has not visited since last October. Think of that.

I have an uncontrollable desire to get on the *V.L.* myself, and catch the Sat. *Home* in Battle and be in Boston Friday the 18th, and come over to Pasque with this letter in my pocket. I would rather do it ten thousand times over than go on the rest of this trip. But I will not back out. You would not like it. If only we do not miss all the boats at Cartwright three weeks hence, or get refused on them all because they are so full, and so be six weeks more instead of four weeks more in getting home. That would be a catastrophe. But there is no use in worrying about that. Only it makes me a bit home sick to linger over this paper and to think how you will handle it and it will see your face and I shall not. I think of Pasque and of all we have there in one another and the children and realize what I am missing. And what I have had there with you. But never mind, this will be over some day.

So often, after long absences, [I came back to] Pasque to be with you or find you. It was so in '87 and then each year 1900 and 1901 and 1902 and 1903 and perhaps, most of all in memory 1893. Though I do not think I have felt such a sense of rest in getting back to you then as in 1900 after I had been at Oberammergau etc. In the sense separation this trip is worse than any of those others.

It is pretty far out of the world up here. When the schooners go back in September and October and no one is left up here except the few 'liveyers' and the 'breeds' and Esquimaux and the occasional Indians who come out to the coast, it must be as if one had gone out of the world.

I cannot help thinking all the time of the homecoming and wondering where I shall meet you again – you will hardly be at Pasque, And most probably in Orange. And I shall not see you until I have been to Cambridge to get my clothes and to see how the house is getting on and all that. In Orange too I shall love to find you there too, it has been the place of many a happy hour coming from long absences.

…But I shall be so glad when the whole thing is over. There will be no thanks deep enough to give if it is once well over with. But I did not mean to write in this way. I meant only to tell you how I love you, and how I long for you and wait for you, and how all my life, but for you, would be like an infinite prolongation and intensification of this Labrador journey…. If only there can be one or more days of quiet with you at Orange or somewhere else after the long restless summer and before the work of the year begins.

Mr. Moore continues to express his loneliness and his love for his wife in the same vein for several pages, concluding:

How can I thank you, bless you, repay you, Bessie? I love you. I love you…

Your husband,
Edward.

JOURNAL ENTRIES

BEGINNING THE JOURNAL
S.S. *Strathcona*, Indian Harbor, Lab. Wed. Aug. 9th.

Excitements began early today. We had not got to bed until midnight. Wood, the London secretary, was going south on the *Virginia Lake* which was expected at any time. Mumford, the doctor, had asked Wood to sleep aboard with us because the hospital was so full. Jones, the secretary, had been told to get the mail ashore for fear the *V.L.* might come in the night. And when he did not do that he was told to give the mail to Wood, at any rate. For fear that he might fail also to do that I went and got my mail out and gave it to Wood.

About half-past one I heard Mumford come aboard from his boat and call Wood saying that the *V.L.* was outside, had been there an hour. He had just sent out the five patients whom he was dismissing in the big boat and wd. take Wood in the canoe if he would make haste. Wood was fairly frightened at the prospect of missing his boat, for he has been here two weeks and would have to remain two more. He got over the side in great excitement. Jones slept the sleep of the unjust. And in the morning there was fierce invective against him for all the mail except my letters had been left behind.

After breakfast Kingman and I took a great climb over the rocks – like mountains – all about and got some good pictures, especially one of an iceberg close in to the shore on the outer side of the island. Kingmans stuff, surgical preparations galore, his thickest clothes and his photographic materials of all sorts sent in May have not yet appeared and he is correspondingly annoyed. On our ramble we picked out a pool high up on the hill which we thought the sun wd. warm so that we could take a bath in it in the afternoon.

After lunch he had the appendical operation on the man whom we brought up from Batteau. He permitted me to see it – a very pretty operation indeed, and the man is doing very well. Then we went up to our pool. But found the bottom of it so covered with a sediment and the whole thing so uninviting – they are all only peat-bogs – that we went down to the sea on the open ocean side and finding a place where the rocks would permit, plunged in – and out. It was the first time I have bathed in Labrador seas, with fifty-four ice bergs in sight – one not a quarter of a mile away. But it was not so bad as you might think and the sun was warm though the breeze was chilling. We repeated the dose four times and then got into our clothes again.

Before we got home we heard the old cannon firing with wh. the natives were preparing to welcome the Governor. From the top of the hill we could see the *Faiona* near the *Strathcona* and the *Scylla*, the man of war lying outside. Grenfell had brought up from Cartwright a boy for the mastoid operation and – much to his own – G's – delight McKenzie, the head man of all the Hudson Bay Trading Co's agents. McKenzie and his friends have been no friends of the Mission and have even been dampening the ardor of former contributors – including even Lord Strathcona.

And here was McKenzie, at Cartwright, in a fit of delerium tremens and all broken down – stomach and everything – from a prolonged go at the scotch. And up he comes on the Governor's boat, sleeps in the Gov's own cabin, disdains the stretcher, but is virtually carried up to the hospital and put to bed in Mumford's room and placed on a regime in which he will get everything but whiskey.

I bought of Mumford an Arctic fox skin, snow white, small but beautiful and very cheap, $5.00.

The Commodore came ashore from the *Scylla* and was conducted round with the Gov. an amusing English swagger with a big monocle and immaculate dress. Consultations ended in this that the Gov. and his sec. were to go aboard the *Scylla* and head straight for Cape Chidley. Grenfell and Kingman were to do the operations and come on on the *Faiona*. And the *Strathcona*, as being so much the slower craft, was to start at 2:30 Thursday morning and try to get to Hopedale, the Moravian Mission for the night. There or somewhere on the way to Nain the *Faiona* will overtake us. I think, the *Strathcona* will hardly go farther than Nain.

But I shall go aboard the *Faiona* and with G. and K. go on until we meet the *Scylla*, or at least as far as Nackvak, the last of the Moravian Missions on this shore. We shall thus see the Moravian Missions and the Esquimaux and some of the magnificent high coast, and that is the main thing. Merely to get to Chidley is a matter of no consequence.

Then we shall practice medicine all the way south – we are making no stop, you see, on the way north – and only plan to get to Cartwright by the 28th or 29th before the eclipse. The *Scylla* and the *Faiona* are both to be there at the eclipse. And the main result of this association with them will be that almost surely the one or the other of them will take Kingman and me aboard, after the eclipse at Cartwright, and get us down to Battle or St. Johns without our having to take the *V.L.* wh. is foul, they say and will be very much crowded. Or else, to go with Miss Edgar's excursion ship wh I would like to avoid.

At all events G. thinks we can surely count on going with the governor on the *Faiona*. I should be very glad if it wd. work out in this way. Otherwise the association with these other craft is something of a bore, and the medical work for these few days is much interfered with. But I have no doubt that the interesting the authorities in everything and the getting through G.'s plans for lighthouses and charts etc. is a full justification. But it has been uncomfortable not knowing from day to day what we shd. do next.

I forgot to say that when it came to the preparations for the appendical operation, the instruments, ether, etc., wh. K. had brought along from Battle cd. not be found anywhere on the ship. K. was in a state – likewise, Sturges – who had vaguest recollections. The old stuff on ship or at Indian had to be used. And then when Grenfell came aboard and K. reported the matter to G. [condemning S. it came out] that he, – G. – had put the things in his own bureau drawer in his private cabin among his clothes and had forgot to tell S. But seemed to think that S. and K. were very foolish for not having searched the ship until they found them. So it goes.

It is too amusing for anything and sometimes exasperating. Such confusion and mess as every locker on the ship presents your [senses with such an odor]. The bear skin is in the locker with ham and bacon we are going to eat. If you lay down an article of clothing it is in the stock for the Mission poor before you can wink your eye. Battle is rolling in medical supplies and Indian has hardly anything etc. etc. The thing will all go to pieces for lack of a competent executive head. But G. would not make such an [executive head for improving] the living, for in any odd moment, and in the most absurd mood, he wd. upset all that the others had been planning and doing for a year.

Meals are at any time from dawn to midnight. This evening when Peter brought his supper down, G. was selling lynx skins to the Commodore in the little cabin wh. serves for everything and it was [some time] before anybody got a bite of grub. And then prayers are held – ten verses of Moody and Sankey.[71] Each verse with a chorus and sung. And a chapter read – and commented on – if it happens to suit him and the conversion of the Jews prayed for,[72] before anybody gets a bite. This happens in the morning when we have been steaming since 2:30 a.m.

[And Grenfell is] out of bed at 8:00 and taking a bath stark naked standing in a [tub] in the middle of the breakfast room – his patients stamping up and down on deck in their hob-nailed boots and occasionally peering down the companion way to see if somebody will not attend to them – when G. howls out something about the invasion of his privacy. And rebukes Peter for bringing down the fish when it is already 8:30 – bkfst at 8:00. Then comes prayers, as I said, and G. says something about maintaining the devout discipline of the Mission boat. It really is the most ludicrous thing you ever saw. It is as much as one can do to keep from roaring with laughter. And he takes it all so seriously.

"They do be shocking – these flies – mosquitos – They never eats a native. But when they finds a Newfoundlander they goes for he."

---

[71] The American evangelist, Dwight L. Moody, and the American gospel singer and composer, Ira David Sankey (the sweet singer of Methodism), on an evangelistic mission to Newcastle-on-Tyne in England in 1873, published a hymn book, *Sacred Songs and Solos*, which incorporated Phillip Phillip's Hymnary, *Hallowed Songs*, plus many additions. It was claimed that this book "Soon found its way into all parts of the British Empire and later on into every Christian land" (William R. Moody, *The Life of Dwight L. Moody*. p. 170f).

[72] The English Prayer Book had a special prayer for the conversion of the Jews, which was especially appointed to be read on Good Friday but could, of course, be used at any time.

NORTH FROM INDIAN HARBOUR
Windsor Harbor, Evg. of Thursday, Aug. 10th.

Beautiful moonlight night. After perfect day in which we have steamed about a hundred and twenty-five miles. Yesterday and today the first wholly clear days we have had at all, on this cruise. But we seem to have run out of the fog. And it is by no means so cold as we found it further up the shore. Ice bergs also smaller though very numerous all day long. Fine northern lights about ten oclock this evening – the first we have seen. Peculiar effect of the constellations – pole star so high in the heavens, c. 55 degrees. Wonderful sunset coloring on these barren cliffs.

"[A man] was brought to G. [who] suggested that he be washed. Then as the story goes, after a quarter of an hour bathing they came to a shirt. And sometime later as they continued, got down to another shirt."

Passed the southernmost of the Moravian Missions, Makkovik Bay late this afternoon, at upper end of great bay. Said to have a fine church etc. Did not go into bay. Shall have chance to go ashore at Hopedale tomorrow. Sturges tells of complete loss of any recollection among the Esquimaux of a time before they were Christians.[73] No folklore except in Scriptural form like the songs etc. of the negroes at the south.

We had a number of men aboard with bad hands so soon as we anchored. But no serious illness among the people on the schooners at this place. Not doing very well with the fish.

We have begun to move inside the great chain of islands wh. extend from here to Chidley. Countless islands all uninhabited. Not one with a tree, all showing tremendous wear at the sea level from the ice in winter and spring – there some times is floe ice here in August. And new ice begins to make before end of September. Icebergs often float for a year or more and

---

[73] There are many pre-Christian legends and stories of the Inuit handed down in various publications, notably, *Them Days: Stories of Early Labrador*, various volumes. Also, Tim Borlase, *The Labrador Inuit*, p. 58f. However, the Christianising of the Inuit certainly undermined the native belief systems as the missionaries did not accept the practices of native spirituality.

increase in size in winter just as they diminish in summer. Countless ducks on the water and scarcely rising as the steamer approaches.

When the *Virginia Lake* made her first trip down in end of May – as far as Indian Harbor she carried 270 men – is allowed to carry 80 – most therefore were on decks in bitter cold. Three men of one crew came to Indian Harbor Hospital, two of them to die of pleurisy, and the third is still in bed very feeble, has nine children at home. A schooner, returning with her load of fish, the seasons catch took one of the bodies a few days ago, the other body is still on the fish stage at Indian lying in salt, with the corded salted fish.

Miss Williams the nurse at Indian has been out here eleven years, has served at each of the three hospitals and is altogether the most capable person I have seen on shore at all in this whole journey. Has seen the whole work created and is almost as devoted to it all as is Grenfell, himself. She is to be at St. Anthony for the winter.

We celebrated the departure from Indian with clean table cloth and napkins, the first since I came on the ship, nearly three weeks. The old ones had come to be like the man I spoke about. There is a laundry at each one of the hospitals and it shd. not be difficult to have supplies at each place.

A MORAVIAN MISSION
Hopedale, Lab. Friday, Aug. 11th.

Steamed from Winsor Harbor between 5:30 and 8.00 this morning. As we came into Hopedale Run saw the *Harmony* lying at anchor. We learned that she had only got in the night before. A large barque with steam, hailing from London, owned by the Society for the Furtherance of the Gospel – The English Moravian Society – which sustains these Labrador Missions though the central spiritual administration is at Herrnhut[74] and though the most of the Brethren are German – only five Englishmen as Moravian Missionaries on this coast.

The *Harmony* is the supply ship. She makes one visit a year. She was unloading already, a huge boat, like a trap-skiff, beside her and a dozen Esquimaux mostly with their white canvas jackets and capuze,[75] bound with fur on their heads. Some in dress more like the settlers – i.e. old sweaters, coats etc. Very marked Esquimaux type of face. The majority of their men are off at the fishing, and in many cases the women are with them – the children stay behind and are cared for at the Mission school. Many of the houses boarded up. Streets in the Esquimaux village full of dogs and children. But there is only about a hundred inhabitants of this settlement and about a hundred more in the area to thirty miles south, seventy miles north and extending back to the trackless forest – the region wh. looks to this Mission for instruction and supplies.

There are two married brothers and one single man stationed here now. School is conducted in Esquimaux this time of year. In the winter when many of the children of the half breed trappers and hunters are left at the Mission school is conducted in English. Services in the church are all in Esquimaux.

---

[74] This word "Herrnhut" means "Lord's Watch." It is located in eastern Germany. The Moravian Society began in Moravia in 1457 as a group of religious reformers. The Society experienced a renewal in the 18th century when given refuge at Herrnhut by a Count Nicholas of Zinzendorf in Saxony. They placed emphasis upon establishing foreign missions and set up the first of a world-wide outreach in Greenland in 1733 (http://www.ualberta.ca).

[75] capuce, a hood

The Mission property looks very attractive as you approach it from the sea. Red painted shingle roofs and the buildings just in the style prevalent in north Germany, even painted to the color of what theirs would be, the stucco and the half timbering. Windows set in same way – French sash. Cupola on church exactly as in a Prussian village. Inside, everything so spotlessly clean, even the deal[76] floors looking like a kitchen table. The floors are sanded whenever the Esquimaux go because of the oil wh. their boots and skin clothing exudes.

In church you might have thought yourself in Germany. A little pipe organ, a large reed organ. In a closet, which the brothers showed us, violins and cellos and a bass viol besides coronets and horns wh. the Esquimaux play at the services. Wooden benches, mostly without backs, oil lamps – until a year ago only candles.

In house, white porcelain stoves and green tile ones too. Sofa place of honour with table pushed against it. Even knickknacks about room so characteristically German. A good many books, partly German and partly English, colored prints, some photographs. In kitchen much tile and shining copper. Bedrooms narrow and like monastic cells off a corridor. Everywhere the red covered down bed covers wh. represent so much misery to one of us.[77] Evident provision for a good deal of hospitality.

At the back connected by a covered gang[78] – there is also a covered gang to church, and to the old school – but not to the larger one built last year – At the back is a long building containing bakery, blacksmith shop, carpenter shop, paint shop and here a storehouse for all things pertaining to boats and to hunting, trapping etc. On the other side of a court the corresponding wing is a storehouse for food – two years supplies – lest the *Harmony* shd. fail to come. And across the fourth side of the quadrangle a woodshed with, I should think, a hundred cords of wood in it. Sometimes they are absolutely buried in snow and sometimes they see not a human being from the outside world for eight months.

---

[76] Deal is a piece of sawn fir or pine wood between 7 and 9 inches wide and 6 feet long and not over 3 inches thick (*The Oxford Dictionary*).

[77] Some people are allergic to bird-down.

[78] Walkway

In almost every window in the dormitory flowers are growing, and at one end of the dormitory was a small greenhouse with many flowers in it. Beyond, a most neat and successful garden, shut in with a high stockade and with sand paths, petunias, portulacca, pansies and a few roses blooming in the open air.

Then, there was a vegetable garden, evidently the object of much care. In each garden a garden house and seats, and outside a grove of trees which the Brethren planted a hundred years ago and wh. with infinite pains has been kept up. No tree thicker than my forearm. But here also paths and seats and at the end a little forest house, just as if it were a wald-spaziergang in north Germany. And we could hardly get the brother to let us see the Esquimaux village so eager was he to show us the gardens and anlage[79] which had cost so much and was so dear to him.

Beside this Park was the graveyard of the native Christians. All the graves bearing little white boards with a number and the name of the dead man or woman, almost always, a Scriptural name – in German – form, Johannes, Elias, Matthias Etc. – this used as a first name and then the Esquimaux name Pomiuk, Okak, etc. as last name. The highest number I saw was 1104, showing that the dead whom the Mission can count as its fruits are many times more numerous than its living force at the present moment.[80]

The graveyard of the brothers is quite a distance away on the side of a little hill, near the site of the old heathen village as it was when the missionaries first came. That was in 1771. The first three missionaries were murdered, and the subsequent ones used the site of their burial place for their own and still do. There lie more than fifty brothers, sisters and little children, the heroes of this work for now 135 years.

The Missions do a good deal of trading with the natives, settlers and even with the Indians from the interior. They sell supplies of every sort and buy

---

[79] Anlage is a word of German origin which means establishing something or preparing something for development.

[80] The first missionary station near Hopedale was built by the Moravian missionary, J.C. Erhardt, in 1752. After he and six of his crew were likely murdered, the effort was discontinued in Labrador until Jens Haven visited the coast in 1764 and a station was built at Nain in 1770. The first permanent station at Hopedale was built in 1782 so there is nearly a century and a quarter of continuous Christian history behind Hopedale in 1905 (Tim Borlase, *The Labrador Inuit*, p. 169f).

furs and fish. The merits of the system are much in dispute. Grenfell thinks the system almost wholly bad. The S. F. G.[81] is organized to trade as well as further the Gospel and it wd. naturally be a pretty difficult task to keep the two purposes in perfect adjustment the one to the other. Methods are antiquated and sometimes advantage is taken.

The two men whom I saw here, however, are very superior men, both young men with little families. Mr. Heddash, a German born in a Moravian Missionary's home in South Africa, working under an English Society in Labrador. Intelligent, natural, devout, but practical and very efficient I should say.

The Esquimaux houses we went into were not one whit more squalid than of some of the English fishermens on Labrador and Newfoundland. The race is dying out, the missionary thought. This largely by the change of food – to flour and molasses and pork instead of blubber etc. the native food. He thought the English fishermen settled on the coast wd. withstand the climate better if they could bring themselves to eat what the Esquimaux used to do instead of the Esquimaux coming to eat what the settlers do.

The vices of civilization have something to do with it for these Christened Esquimaux are astonishingly pure and almost perform…. But any indoor life undermines them. And when any contagious disease breaks out among them it is apt to make a pretty clean sweep. This is true not only of small pox or diphtheria but even of measles and grippe.

Altogether, I think I have never spent a more interesting hour.

---

[81] The Society for the Furtherance of the Gospel

GRENFELL'S MISFORTUNE
On the Way to Nain, Sat. 12th Aug.

Grenfell has had a hard and humiliating experience and one which I think he will be slow to forget. While we lay at Fannies Harbor, on the south side of Cape Harrigan[82] waiting for him, Sturges and I climbed to the top of the Cape, part of the way over glacier. Wonderful view, especially inland – scores of islands, deep bays and inlets, far away great mountains. Fishermen have had very poor luck – only about a hundred quintals representing the whole summer work of sixteen men. Their eagerness to know how men were doing elsewhere, where fish was being caught etc. was truly pitiable.

Traps never in water more than a couple of hours at a time on account of ice, though fish came here on the 8th of July. Floe ice only disappeared from mouth of the harbor last Sunday, viz. Aug. 6th. They could hardly change their location however at this late date, good berths for traps being taken in most places, and there are free fights and litigation over it enough already. Large part of the magistrates work in summer is in the settling of such disputes. And then the peoples little all is put in plant here, stagings, tilts, or sod houses to live in, and all their gear could hardly be moved and set up again before the season is over.

Presently, the *Faiona* came in, and Grenfell and Kingman came aboard. The plan now was that we were to go into Davis Strait, to the Hudson Bay Co's agency for wood to save our coal. Go on to Nain and get 10 tons of coal wh. G. put there last year, and then work slowly south, caring for the sick, till Grenfell overtook us. For he proposed to go on toward the north to meet the Governor as he came back on the *Scylla*, and take him in to visit the main places of interest. K. thought it rather strange that G. shd. [do this]. But after all this business with the government people has come up later and is important, touches some things he has been waiting for for years. The Minister of Marine and Fisheries is aboard the *Faiona* etc.

---

[82] north from Cape Harrison

And at latest we were all to round up at Cartwright on the 27th. And the Minister and the Captain had promised on the afternoon of the 30th to take Kingman and me aboard and leave us at Battle Harbor. So all seemed very fair. The only thing wh. G. seemed uneasy about, and the skipper thought they were putting upon Grenfell, was the fact that the man who has piloted the *Faiona* up to Cape Harrigan declared his contract at an end, declared he had no competent knowledge beyond that, and so G. was in full and undivided responsibility. The ship is so much bigger than the *Strathcona* that the courses which the latter uses are not always available for her and G. hardly knows the others.

Once outside the Cape we swung off to the west to go through the Strait, and they went to the north for the outside course. We had set sail and were bowling along under both sail and steam, then came up a squall and for a time we were busy. Meantime we suddenly became aware that the *Faiona* was following us, as if to go through the Inlet, too. She passed us, running very fast, and bantering us on being too slow.

Just before the group of huts which constitute the Hudson Bay Station were reached the *Faiona* veered from the course and went hard aground. She was going nine knots an hour and rammed the shoal in great shape, ran high up at the bow and then the bow settled off into deeper water, but she remained hanging about amid ships. Fortunately, it was only sand or mud, though there were rocks all around. And fortunately the tide was nearly half down. But as it continued to fall, she came out of water till she showed two feet of copper and her screw was half out of water, and slowly careened until masts and funnel had a bad list.

Indians, Esquimaux, halfbreeds and later the agent swarmed out. All shook their heads, and we were very blue. Grenfell was all broken up, almost broken down. Had had the ship in charge not yet two hours. The land lubbers on her were frightened. The Minister of Marine was at least dubious as to whether he ought to have brought her. The wise cursed Grenfell for having, in the mood and whim of a moment, abandoned the outside course and everybody dumped all blame and responsibility on G. of course. Even our own skipper said it came from taking a responsibility wh. he ought never to have taken in the world.

We anchored along side of them. By this time it was growing dark and raining in sheets and the wind rising. I do not think there was much sleep on either ship. She must be pulled off at high tide, about 4:00 a.m., if she wd. come. If not, she must be lightened – and that wd. have been no small task with only their four boats and our two – and then the attempt made again at 4:00 p.m. If we failed utterly it looked as if we might have to steam to Chateau – three days – in order to telegraph to St. Johns for tugs – wh. wd be a week in coming. And then what condition might she be in and how about the eclipse and our own connection home etc. etc.

Toward morning, it ceased to rain, and at 3:30 we got to work again. She put out an anchor and a grapnel from her stern with lines toward the channel, and we gave her a wire cable, and when all was ready, and she moving full speed astern and winding on her winch we went ahead full speed. Five times we tried it and it seemed as if something, somewhere would have to part. But at 5:10 off she came and we towed her stern first into deep water. They made an examination to see if she was leaking and signalled that she was not, and that they were off to get through the Inlet with high water.

Five minutes after, and just as we were anchoring, they signalled us again to wait. G. came aboard and said that the people on board were in such a funk they would not go through the Inlet except in the wake of our boat. So we shd. leave the wood and put them through to Paul's Island on the open sea and then put back to Nain, the Moravian Mission, for Sunday.

It must have been very humiliating for G. and it bodes no pleasant residence on board of the *Faiona* for him for the next ten days.[83] And this is what we are doing now, going through this forty miles of narrow tortuous channel full of rocks and…countless islands, the yacht following with her bowsprit almost glued to our wake, and old Bartlett grumbling that he has to take

---

83 Grenfell describes this incident and its consequences in *A Labrador Doctor* (p.192). He also describes several other groundings and close calls. He was on the *Sir Donald* when she ran aground on Caribou Island near Battle Harbour. He was steering the *Strathcona* 2 when she struck a rock and was abandoned, briefly. He was in peril when several other vessels went ashore in a gale at Indian Tickle.

responsibility of two ships at once. But they do not propose to run aground in our absence. In this particular case they would never have got off with their own steam in the world. And how easily it might have happened that we were miles away. Once in the open sea, they will feel better.

I am sorry we could not land at the Davis Strait Station today for there are scores of Indians from the interior who have come out for supplies. They are full blooded Indians of the wandering tribes of the mountains[84] in the Hudsons Bay territory and are rarely seen by white men. There are only men here, their wives and children having been left eleven days journey away, they say, and they are all on the verge of starvation. They say they can never remember a year when there were so few deer, so little game of any sort. They have comparatively few furs. But they must have food.

The worst of it is that the Company's supply ship, the *Pelican*, went on a reef between Battle and Indian Harbors about three weeks ago on her way north. Was badly broken, and finally was towed all the way to St. Johns taking all her precious cargo with her – why they did not land it and let some other vessels bring it up, I do not know. Meantime flour is $18.00 a barrel at the Station and almost none at that price. Everything in proportion. And if the winter sets in before the supplies arrive there will be very many Indians and Esquimaux who will not see the spring.

I never saw such Indians as those who put off in their boats. And there was not so very much that we could give them, something like a square meal for the few who came aboard. The halfbreeds impress me most pitifully of all, so often they are degenerate, one way or another. One old man came out in a miserable canoe of his own make last night, the very picture of lonely woe, and incapacity.

[84] These were the Montagnais Innu, known by some of the English settlers as "Mountaineers."

MORE DIFFICULTIES ON THE JOURNEY
Black Island, 20 Miles N.E. of Nain,
on *Strathcona*, Sunday, Aug. 13th.

Spent a miserable day yesterday through Grenfells indecision and the evident breaking down of his plans. We led the way for more than half the day, their bowsprit almost over our stern. Then, our air pump broke down. We hauled off and explained to them supposing that they would go on without us. Instead of that Grenfell proposed to tow us, so that we should remain together. A line was got out and our men went to work to repair the engine.

Then Grenfell explained that he wanted us to go with them as far as Fords Harbor. Later, he changed his mind and decided we should go to Black Island, the edge of the open sea, and outside the island runs. Meantime, so soon as the fog shut down on us they being in the lead, they stopped moving and finally sent aboard for our skipper to come aboard the *Faiona* to show them the way. And incidentally it was said that we should go as far as Okak, the northmost of the Moravian Stations and a hundred miles from here. That was vetoed by our engineers saying that we had not coal enough – this very days towing us about having taken us far beyond Nain where our only coal lay.

K. and I were in a state of mind for we thought it doubtful, if we went as far north as Okak whether we could get back in time for the eclipse without steaming every day, and leaving no margin for the bad weather we are fairly sure to get.

Finally it was proposed to take our skipper as well as Grenfell on the bridge of the *Faiona* and leave us here for a week or ten days without anybody who even knew enough to get us to Nain to get our coal, much less to get us away in case of failure in any way to connect with them. This plan…K. and I resented, not to put it too strongly. I do not know if G. had really thought it through in all its bearings. It seems incredible that he should have attempted to enforce it. But one or two people who have come up here have had grim experiences when it suited him. Young Bond was left for six weeks at Inglee at the lumber camp and finally escaped by a schooner.

However, it was finally settled that the skipper was to come aboard again with us, as he flatly refused to act as pilot of the other and take the responsibility wh. G. has so lightly taken. Then it was decided to take old man Ford from here as a pilot. But when we got here old man Ford was gone south and then there was more debating.

I honestly think if there had been room on board the *Faiona* we should have been forced to go aboard of her and the question reopened with our skipper and he almost or quite forced to go at G's command. It was painfully evident that the *Faiona*'s company had lost every particle of confidence in G's piloting, justly or unjustly I cannot say. And I think it was evident that G. had considerably lost confidence in himself to do the thing he had felt he could do so easily.

I suspect that if old man Ford had been here G. would have been excused from further attendance on the govt. party. As it was, he had to go, and they had to take him as pilot. At six p.m. they got under way for the run to Davis Island, three hours farther north, and they will surely run all day Sunday for they are a day behind their schedule with the *Scylla* and the governor, all owing to the unwise attempt to go through the runs instead of going outside at once they left Fannies Harbor.

We settled down to spend the night and Sunday in this bleak forbidding place. There are two houses on the shore and two schooners in the Harbor. I shall hold service twice in one of the houses. They seemed very glad to have us. It rained all night and toward morning blew hard. We had to get out another anchor, and there is a choppy sea, even in close to the shore. The cabin is very comfortable. We have a fire in the little stove and plenty to read.

And this morning we had trout for breakfast, brought from the shore. One of these trout was thirteen inches long. We are right at the foot of the great Keiglapeit [Kiglapait] range of mountains wh. here comes right out to the sea. If only the clouds lift so that we can see them before we leave.

They are said to be very fine. But it is settling in for a very rainy day and the wind has gone down.

I cannot deny that it is infinite relief to have got rid of the governmental party, and it [might even be] a relief to be rid of Grenfell so long as he is in this frame of mind which this confusion of his plans has brought on. I thought he looked last night as if he would have given a good deal to be out of this scrape. And the worst of it is, that after what has happened, and in the resentful and distrustful frame of mind in wh they all are avoiding him, I doubt if he has gained anything by this whole move.

I suspect that he is further from the cordial support of the politicians etc. Before, he was known to them only as the idol of the Labrador shore, and a force, more or less unknown to them, wh wd have to be reckoned with. Now they will think they know him and have seen his work – they know not, of course – but they will say they have unmasked him, that he is not what he is cracked up to be, that he is…all of which is grossly untrue.

But yet this is true. That he is often very over confident. That he meddles with a great many things wh he knows very little about, and has a thousand schemes rather than any fixed solid well drawn and adhered to plan. That he has no organizing talent, and sometimes comes to grief. And they have seen him just at one of these times.

ANOTHER MORAVIAN MISSION
Nain, Labrador. Monday, August 14th.

Got away from Black Island about 6 this morning and were at Nain at 9:30. Very beautiful mountains and cliffs on the way. Very cold, almost like November or early December at home. Bright sunlight early in the day but soon overcast and with strong to high wind. Landed at Nain where, so soon as we cast anchor the Esquimaux swarmed out in their boats. Hired ten of them to help get coal and water.

Coal is Scotch coal brought here by the *Harmony* last year and was put in a shed not very tight. Shed filled with snow in winter, later snow melted, and now, 14th August, the coal pile is frozen hard as a rock. We got seven tons by the aid of the pick axe, lightered it out to the ship in scows and hoisted it aboard in big old puncheons – a hard piece of work from beginning to end. Water was brought out in the same way, a thousand gallons, in puncheons on the scows and put in tanks by lines of Esquimaux with buckets. When it came to paying them at least twice as many claimed to have worked on the job as the skipper had employed.

We met the two chief men here at the Mission, Bishop Martin and Brother Schmitt, and were shown through gardens and greenhouse and little strip of forest with carefully laid out walks. Flowers were really wonderful when you consider what an amount of loving labor they must have cost. I do not think the Brothers would be more grateful for anything than for flower seeds sent to them. Vegetable gardens quite as remarkable – with all things which will ripen in a short summer. In every garden a garden house – screened from mosquitoes – seats along the paths in the forest, and such pride in this whole part of the plan – in proportion to the labor it had cost, the rarity of such a thing in this part of the world, and the Germans love of such things. But the mosquitoes – particularly in the forest – were worse than I have ever seen them anywhere. Faces and hands were all bloody when we came into the house.

House is very like the one at Hopedale only bigger. Built about 70 years ago, much of it brought from Germany, porcelain stoves etc. Very comfortable indeed. Spotlessly clean. School, shops, Church all very much as at Hopedale. Esquimaux village very much larger – about a hundred houses.

Martin, the Bishop, is a Saxon, and his wife is also Saxon, but born in a Moravian Missionary home in South Africa. They always speak German. In fact Martin finds it rather difficult to speak in English. They have had eight children, four are dead and buried here – one killed by the dogs – three are in Germany at school.

Frau Martin far superior to her husband, a really remarkable woman, it seemed to me, so kind and hospitable, so simple and devoted. Schmitt is the son of a Moravian Missionary in Greenland, educated in Germany, resided long in London, and married an English wife – a man far superior to the Bishop, and well worth remembering. Fine little boy, about 8 who must go back with the *Harmony* a few weeks hence to the Brothers school at Fullneck in Yorkshire, England. Another little boy about 3 and a baby just a week old – so that we did not see Mrs. Schmitt. Must send both families something for Christmas. A young man, Hilby, a German, unmarried, as storekeeper and a young Englishman named Heath, constitute at present the family.

The storekeeper who had been here for some years and of whom they all seem to have been very fond had been growing very eccentric for some time, and occasioning them many questions and perplexities, finally went raving crazy. They had to confine him and latterly from three to eight men had to watch him, and hold him. He was sent away last week on the *Virginia Lake* to St. Johns to be put in the asylum.

Sadly enough a rather attractive young woman named Frl Grundemann, came out on the *Harmony* to marry him. She arrived one day before the *V. L.* left with him for St. J. She did not see him at all he was so violent. She goes back with the *Harmony* to her family in Germany a few weeks hence. As Frau Martin said, it was the sadder because they had known and loved one another long. While often the brides sent out by the Directory have not even seen the men for whom they are designated.

We spoke German most of the time. They all seemed delighted to have the chance. We took dinner and again supper with them. Potted reindeers flesh for dinner – they mean caribou of course – and again smoked caribou for supper, also a kind of wurst – caribou and pork together. Green beans for dinner out of their own garden, also lettuce, and in the evening rhubarb – think of it – for us on such a cruise as this when we never see a green thing. Cooking so good, too, so unlike the filth and sameness of everything on the boat. Had a good Hamburg cigar after dinner, visited the stores, and was most interested in the kind of things which such a post-traders place has to carry, everything for fishing, trapping, hunting, boats, even guns, ammunition, clothing, bedding, household utensils beside foods.

It is a great great pity we cd. not have been here for Sunday as we planned instead of being hung up at Black Island. For yesterday was their Communion. As it was described to me they still observe the old custom of the Unitas Fratrum, the men kissing all the other men and the women all the other women after the rite. I believe the brothers also kiss the brothers and the sisters the sisters as they sit on either side of the pulpit. But they do not deem it necessary to kiss all the Esquimaux – that would be something of an ordeal – But the form of service and the music and the preaching etc. I shd. greatly have enjoyed.

As it was, that loss was somewhat made up to us by the fact that we were allowed to attend a funeral of two men who had died the night before of pneumonia – two others are very ill. The funeral was at 5:00 in the Church and pretty much the whole community was there. Even the loading of coal ceased for the time and the Esquimaux came up just as they were, at the ringing of the bell.

The Bishop read a little discourse wh. I noticed he had written in fine pen and ink notes and the liturgy for burial was gone through with – there were at least six places in it where the people took part in Chorals, sung to old German Choral music much of wh. I know. Equally, at the grave – whither almost the whole congregation adjourned – there was solemn reading from the liturgy and singing. Here also, the mosquitoes were almost beyond endurance.

The brothers gave us a most interesting book on the history of the Moravian Mission in Labrador – and it would take me a day to write out the interesting things they told me about the life on the coast and the vicissitudes of their work. The touring in the winter is the most extraordinary part of it. Schmitt made a tour last winter to Nackvak, 149 miles, with 2 men and 15 dogs in 14 hours.

In the funeral service, I noticed that the numerals were in German. I asked why. Martin said that the Esq. could not count beyond 10, which they called a half man, viz., his 10 fingers, while 20 – his 10 toes added – made a whole man – forty is 2 men, 60 is three men etc. thus 75 would be 2 ½ [*sic*] men and five.[85] The translators of Bible, liturgy etc. found this too cumbrous and introduced German numerals.

---

[85] 75 would be 3 ½ men and five.

SOUTH FROM NAIN
Tuesday, Aug. 15th

It has blown half a gale all day and at times rained hard. We went up to the Mission to call and render our thanks, got away just before dinner, brought away two Esq. women, each with a baby, and two boys, to go down to join their husbands at Fords Harbor where we are lying tonight.

The women carry their babies in their hoods and will do all kinds of work without the baby falling out. Schmitt said he had seen a woman lay a perfectly naked baby on a bank of snow. Tales of his about the Esq. gorging when he has food and his sleeping when he has leisure. And about his endurance of cold etc. Jolly happy, always. But foully dirty, curious as little children. Kingmans magic tricks etc. called forth their amazement and infinite hilarity. Almost none of them ever learn to swim.

I bought a white seal skin and a few little mementoes, Labradorite, a model kayak etc. Here at Fords Harbor, Pauls Island, we are in shelter. But it is a howling gale outside and as cold as winter. One has the uneasy sense how easy it wd. be to be shut in at any time now by the setting in of the winter, and never get away from here until next July. Of course that is nonsense just yet. But any moment after the middle of Sept. it is always possible. The *V. L.* will not come again now because of the eclipse. There will be a Christmas mail – arriving here about end of January – and then not another until July or August 1906.

Tales Of Ice And Foxes
Tuesday and Wednesday, Aug. 15th and 16th.

Nothing of note. Went to House Island and Quircks Tickle, then in through the Rattle to Davis Inlet. Anchored opposite the Hudson Bay Company's station Wednesday evg. and near the spot of the *Faionas* going aground last week.

Wednesday and Thursday beautiful days, the first except Thursday and Friday of last week which we have had in the whole cruise. The medical practice offered nothing new or worthy of note. The Rattle was very beautiful, like a Norwegian Fiord as I imagine these. Have come on today, Thursday, by three or four stations, and are anchored for the night at the Lance Ground beyond Fannies Harbor.

Had a good chance to see the Indians today at Davis Inlet, or at least to see some of them – those of last week are gone away in despair. The trader still has no supplies. But ten or a dozen Indians – Nascaupies are here from eleven days journey back in the forest. Interesting people. So much superior to the Esquimaux. An old man, his two sons and nephew and the wife of the eldest son and another woman we had aboard and gave them as much as they could eat.

No one of them except the father had even seen a steamboat or engine. But for that matter no one of them has ever seen a horse. They were very thin and gaunt. But had brought out very little fur, and look forward to the next winter with no little apprehension. They were all Roman Catholics. One woman wore a large white metal crucifix. The old man could talk very good English.

The man Guy, the Hudson Bay Companys agent, seemed quite a decent sort of a fellow. But what a life, especially for his wife and two children.

Going out we took with us an old Brigus master fisherman a friend of the Captains, who is having particularly bad luck with the fishing. Has five schooners and almost sixty men all told in his employ but has caught little or nothing thus far. He has his stages and houses here and cannot very well move.

He told a wonderful story of two of his men. Off twelve miles to sea lies a particularly barren rock called The Farmyard, – it must be in bitter irony – but it has always been a great place for fish. When he got down here the 5th of July with his crews, he sent two men in a skiff out there to pre-empt the good places – berths they call them – they had ten days food, their traps etc. and the schooner was to follow them. There was not a pan of floe ice anywhere to be seen but beautiful clear sea and sky.

Five days later when the schooner was on her way over there, the wind changed, the ice came in, the schooner brought up fifty miles up the coast having all she could do to save herself. When fifteen days had passed Spracknell gave the two men up for lost. But a day or two later they came in having dragged the boat – a good sized trap skiff – over ice whenever ice was solid enough and pushed her through when it was open water. It was bitter cold, dense fog, and they were almost starved.

The ice cleared away only last week. This is the reason why they have no fish. The fish have been here all the time in great numbers, but the nets could not be kept down. In an unlucky moment when we were here last week somebody told Grenfell that the fishermen here had twelve young foxes – we already have four aboard. He told the skipper to buy them when we should come back. This we have just done at $5.00 a head, grays, most of them. The men brought them aboard in two bags, and we put them in the old cage while our four wh. are fairly tame run about the deck. Tomorrow we must have a new cage made at Hopedale.

But the odor of the whole front portion of the ship is getting to be something fierce. The zoo is nothing to it. And all the deck aft is loaded with some 20 cords of wood to go to Indian Harbor for the Hospital. So there is nothing for the passengers to do but climb to the crosstrees and sit as near as possible to the masthead trying to get a breath of fresh air.

The boat is so small and was already so filthy and so crowded with every thinkable and unthinkable thing, and the service is so inadequate to the doing of the work already necessary that the discomfort is real and not wholly imaginary. One of the twelve foxes got away in the scrimmage on shore before they were got in their bags. And if some of them do not die in their close confinement before they get to St. Anthony I am no prophet.

I am thinking with vast amusement of Miss Edgar's extravagant advertisement of her Labrador party – viz. that at Cartwright – besides seeing the eclipse – Dr. Grenfell and the *Strathcona* would join her party – I think I see the fine ladies etc. of that party now coming aboard to visit the *Strathcona* and being driven over the rails again by the odor of the foxes – wh. is more like that of skunks than anything I have yet met. We think of running up a yellow flag and putting a man at the rail to say that we have fifteen cases of small fox aboard the hospital ship and no one can come aboard.

WELCOME AT HOPEDALE
Aug. 18th

After an abjectly miserable night with the fifteen foxes scratching and fighting and careening round in the moon-light over our heads – the four that we had before had been let loose on the deck and the new ones put in their old box because these last were so wild – and we struck, moved the cages aft over the rudder gear where the odor could float off in clouds. Poor old Bill cleaned up the deck in groans and maledictions.

It was a glorious day. The fourth, I think it is, wh. we have had on this whole summer cruise. So foggy and cold it has been. We reached Hopedale just before noon. Went ashore to call on the brothers while the men got drinking water in the casks and a box to make an additional fox cage. Nothing would do but we must see the gardens and the walks through the sad wizened little trees again. And we must stay to dinner. Such a good table. Caribou meat and spinach with eggs and lettuce salad etc. So nicely cooked and so cleanly served.

Mr. Lenz and his wife who was born here at Hopedale – she is the daughter of Br. Jannasch of Makkovik. Educated in Germany, they have two babies, and Hettasch who does all the medical work though he is not regularly qualified as a physician. His wife is a pleasant little woman from Neuwild on the Rhine. The storekeeper is an Englishman – Goleby. Lenz will have to go to Nain to take the place of the man who has gone insane.

At dinner it came out that Hettash was going tomorrow to Double Island to the Esquimaux Colony to spend Sunday, to look after his flock there. It is about 25 miles. We gave him and his Esquimaux boat man a tow over to the Island and Hettach came aboard. He took supper with us and also spent the night and had breakfast, though I was almost ashamed to have him, the contrast of his table and ours was so great, especially in point of cleanliness.

When we got to the islands we had a regular siege of patients so that we never got off the boat until half past seven and even then spent our time going from house to house among the Esquimaux to see the sick and leave them medicines. Hettach wanted to see and hear everything about the medical practice of course. I was most interested to see the inside of the Esquimaux houses.

In the house of one Manasseh one of the Chief of the Hopedale men, we found five sick persons out of eighteen – they all lived in two rooms – and had built a sort of a shed for Hettach to put up in when he goes over for Sundays. One young man, Manasseh's son-in-law, I think will die. He is far on the way with consumption.

Hettach showed us with great pride and joy a little church with red shingle roof like the Mission buildings, all so neat without and within wh. the Esquimaux have built with their own labor and at their own expense – it was at their own motion entirely and the old man Manasseh was the chief mover in it. It is the first church wh. the Mission Esquimaux have built for themselves and of their own suggestion.

In it was a reed-organ made in Carlsrule which the *Harmony* brought out and wh. the men brought over to the islands in an open boat. Every stick of timber, every board and shingle, every nail came over in the same way, for the island is absolutely barren. Grenfell gave them some of the lumber from his mill at Canada Bay.

The Hopedale Esquimaux have had their huts etc. for summer fishing here for many years and were unwilling to go on any longer without a church. They spend about four months out of every year here and take their wives and children and dogs all over in their open boats. They cannot even leave their dogs in Hopedale for nobody would undertake the feeding of them. Whenever fish are being caught they live on the refuse.

We went into the little church with a lantern. Hettach played a little and there gathered a score of men, women and children to see what we were doing. We all sang. When we came out, the whole northern heavens was resplendent with the beautiful white light of the Aurora. It was the only fine display which I have yet seen. So constantly have our nights been rainy or foggy. In the afternoon also we had seen the only whale which I have yet seen. It was quite close by us, though not a very large one, the skipper said.

On the way back we stopped on a Newfoundland schooner to see a girl who was aboard as cook and was sick in the hold. Such filth, stench, desolate discomfort, denial of every proper condition for human existence I have rarely seen. There were nine men on the schooner which was a craft of less than a hundred tons burden. She earned the skipper said, probably thirty or thirty five dollars wages over and above her keep for the whole four months cruise, even five months sometimes. The Esquimaux huts were palaces compared with the hold of that ship. The crew had had poor luck and were sour and disappointed. Altogether, it was one of the forlornest visits which we have made at all.

The Esquimaux on the other hand were reported as doing very well. Their costume, especially of the women was often very curious. Old cast off clothes of ladies in the states pieced out with the white hoods, seal skin pantaloons and skin boots of the native. Only the children were in pure native costume wh. is so picturesque. In winter, they wear only Esquimaux clothes.

MAKKOVIK ON SUNDAY
Saturday, Aug. 19th.

Visited the two Turnaviks and brought up at the Mission at Makkovik for the Sunday. At the upper end of a narrow bay about 9 miles from the sea on edge of the forest. Wind still evening and mosquitoes fearful. Brother Townley came off and spent evening with us. Sunday it was positively hot in this little pocket. Not a breath of wind, later, what there was was off shore and the mosquitoes were ten times worse than ever. It was a miserable day, to be sure, and we were sorry we had not remained at E. Turnavik with Captain Bartlett and his people there.

In the morning there came aboard a man who turned out to be the servant at the Mission, who asked for gramophone records. Said he had had the machine for two years and last year the Dr. had promised to bring him some new records. Particularly he wanted <u>sacred</u> ones – hymns etc. The catalogues wh. he had had contained no entries of <u>sacred</u> records. We got up the box and ultimately dug up Grenfells machine and tried the records, that the man might hear them.

This procedure we had cause to rue for when they got to going, our own boys from the crew and some who came off from the shore, they never knew when to stop and the thing became a more utter nuisance than even the mosquitoes had been. Finally when it had drifted, this concert, from, Onward Christian Soldiers and Gauls, Holy City to the vulgarest minstrel show songs, we put a stop to it as unworthy of the ship and certainly not according to Grenfell's wish for a Sunday.

The man who probably earns less than a hundred dollars a year in cash took four records at prices of 75 cents and a dollar each and at night he came back and got one more. He took Gauls, Holy City, Onward Christian Soldiers, Yield Not to Temptation, a shabby minstrel parody of The Sewanee River and a ventriloqual imitation of the riot in a bird store when a hand organ played in the street.

To think that all that is represented to us by a street-band, a concert, the theatre, or opera, orchestra, minstrel show and even declamation, humoristics etc., not to say church choirs, organs etc. is represented to these wilds by the accursed grind and wheeze and hum and titter of a gramophone, imitating in this forlorn way something wh. can be only an object of imagination to one who has never been away from these shores.

I was reminded that Kingman told that when he and Grenfell were on their way down on the *Faiona* they stopped at Long Tickle to put ashore a woman named Morgan who had brought down a little girl to be operated on at Indian Harbor. They stumbled up to a house in the dead of night, found the whole fishing crew, ten or a dozen of them sleeping on the floor like sardines in a box. Asked what he Grenfell, could do for them, whether they had any sick, or anything of that sort. Some man from the darkness replied, No, no, Dr. but if you have got any gramophone records we shd. like to have some.

At the Makkovik Church were few Esquimaux and Townley preached in English and I followed him. There was a small audience anyway, most of the people being at the fisheries. There are but few at best. Only four families here the year round. The house and church on the other hand are the biggest on the coast. It seems as if the planting of the station in this place had surely been a mistake. Some old lady in England, I believe, gave the money for the church and insisted upon its being a new station etc.

Townley and his wife are alone here now. But Perrits wife and two little children are with them while Perrit is gone with the *Harmony* to St. Johns. When he comes back the Perrits go to Killinek to the new station at Cape Chidley. Mrs. Perrit and Mrs Townley are sisters. The Townleys have one child. Townley was long stationed at Ramah and Hebron in the north and had many most interesting stories to tell of excursions on the ice with the Esquimaux, walrus hunting etc. and of journeys with the dogs, of the habits of dogs and Esquimaux etc. He seemed a man well fitted for this sort of thing. But as a missionary he seemed to me far inferior to the Germans who we have seen at Nain and Hopedale.

MOSQUITOES, FOXES AND MORE PATIENTS
Monday Morning, Aug. 21st.

We have come out to Makkovik Islands, getting away at 4:00 o'clock because the night had been so hot and the mosquitoes so bad nobody got much sleep. And here it is cold again and there are seventy-odd ice bergs in sight, in the glittering sunlight. Such a change.

We had a bad time with the foxes yesterday. There are too many for our close quarters for them and if we do not get them to Indian pretty soon and put them on shore, some of them will die. One of them had fits and one got overboard and in the middle of the night one was found in the after cabin among the men who turned out and gave him a chase. They and the dogs raced over the deck all night and added their share to the impossibility of sleep. The state of the deck can better be imagined than described.

Old Bill is a long suffering man. I do not believe that any sailor is bound to do what he does on this deck. And if he shd. strike and leave us we shd. be in a fix. For I am certain that there is not another soul aboard who would do what he does. Bill says "I bin cleaned out dat fox box. It do be shocking. I bin in courageous turmoil my time but dat is de most tremendous smell dat ever I witnessed. I buried dead harses to de mines, but dis bi de head smell dat ever I seed."

K. took a photograph of a very large ice-berg with an arch in it and an opening through above the arch, very rotten above and liable to fall any minute, so that we dare not put out a boat to lie alongside to measure by. But it was certainly a hundred feet high.

Captain speaking of extravagance says – An Esquimaux in Hopedale, he haves a horgan in his 'ut, it might be an 'armonium, but I think it is a horgan. Peter always says, Huskymaw.

The floyes is bad. – Cotton masks and engine-oil smudge is worse.

Esquimaux stories of Townley about the phrase, bad job. – His account of the two insane men who traversed the coast, the one from Quebec and the other from St. Johns, enduring things that no sane man could ever have endured in the world. The fright of the lonely women and children when they came. The kindness of the Esquimaux to them everywhere, giving one of them a laconic note – "He eats anything."

Aionamat says the Esquimaux for anything which cannot be remedied, almost as the Mohammedan says, Kismet.[86]

How is the fish, down along? or, How is the fish to the north? says the Newfoundlander as he comes over the side.

Today we visited in Long Tickle a halfbreed woman who had one breast removed for cancer two years ago, an entirely successful piece of work but who refused to come with us to Indian today, to have the other removed tho K. thinks it is high time.

Saw Mary Anne Anderson a little girl of eleven eldest of seven the youngest a week old. Mary Anne was keeping the whole establishment, sick mother, new baby, busy father, all children and nine dogs.

Looked at a caribou hide for study floor. But it is wrong time of year all the hair comes out. Counted 174 icebergs around horizon this 21st day of August, and we almost perished with heat yesterday. Saw several grampuses, huge big things, they go as high as 800 or 900 lbs in weight.

"Erring-'awgs,[87] the Newfoundlanders say.

As we lay at Ragged Islands delayed by the great number of patients, we sighted the *Virginia Lake* and soon had our mail. Letters from B. nos[88] 3 and 4 of July 26th and Aug. 1st. Mothers Aug. 8th, May July 31st. It seems as if one or even two of Bessie's must have been kept back some

---

[86] Moore is comparing the word "aionamat" in the Inuktitut language to the Islamic term "kismet" which, according to *The Concise Oxford Dictionary*, means destiny, a predetermined course of events. It derives from the Arabic word "qismah" meaning either the will of Allah or one's lot or fate in life. The native reaction to those who spoke or acted in an abnormal way was that the Creator made them as they were for a purpose and they were to be accepted and treated kindly.

[87] dolphins, also known as herring hogs

[88] numbers

way. They are so incredibly stupid and careless here. But even as it is I know that things must have been all well up to Aug. 8th wh. is only 2 weeks ago. Such a famine I have never suffered, not a word or sign of any sort have I had since August 1st at Battle Harbor.

ANXIETY ABOUT THE PASSAGE HOME
Tuesday, Aug. 22nd.

At Ragged Islands before we left this morning a Welsh barquentine with salt, came in and in doing so, struck on a ledge with a crack which resounded even to our ears. Carried away her stern entirely and tore a big hole in her false bow. She swung off into deep water and there was scurrying to see if she were aleak. But she appeared to hold water, so they set about her repairs there.

We got some photographs of the queer place and got away about 10:00 a.m. and steamed straight to Indian Harbor. Hard squall in the afternoon with sheets of rain and towering high sea. Quiet again before we got to Indian. Wonderful aurora at night. At Indian found the man operated on for appendicitis up and about work. The old woman from Batteau whose clothes, all except what she was carried ashore in, Sturges forgot and carried with us to the north, is never going to need them. She is dying of tuberculosis condition of the bowels.

Mrs. Swarfield had come up from Cartwright to be operated on by K. She brought Cartwright news. The *Virginia Lake* does not wait for eclipse passengers, but goes right back at end of this week, passing here Friday. She will not be here again for more than two weeks. Miss Edgars excursion has fallen through and does not come at all. Canadian Govt. expedition goes to Rigolet and not to Cartwright. So that our sole reliance is the *Faiona* or to take the *V. L.* this week. This I am inclined to do but K. hesitates, and feels more sure of our reliance on the *Faiona* than I do. We must debate it. I shall send mail by the *V. L.* on Friday at any rate, part of this journal. But I am very loath to run even the chance of getting left. And I do not like the having only one string to the bow. Must debate it tomorrow.

PUTTING IN TIME
Wednesday, Aug. 23rd.

Bright and beautiful day but with high wind and cold. Ship being painted and cleaned. Kingman had two operations. Took long walk and climb on this and neighboring islands, using Mumford's canoe to get from one to another. The father of Jarrett, the trader here, is the original of Jagger in, *Dr. Luke*. He died in St. Johns penitentiary for barratry. Not any love lost between him and Grenfell.

MORE CONCERNS ABOUT RETURNING HOME
Wednesday evening, Aug. 23rd.

The captain offered today to take us in the *Strathcona* to Cartwright, leaving twenty four hours after the *Virginia Lake* left here, if we could find that she went to Rigolet. So long we could wait for the *Faiona*. But he was quite clear that if the *F.* was not here by that time, it was because some change of plan had been entered upon and we ran the greatest risk of not getting away from Cartwright until the tenth of Sept. and not home until the 22nd or 23rd. That settles it I think, for I cannot possibly be so late with all my opening terms work to prepare.

If the *Virginia Lake* does not stop at Rigolet, then we must take her here. And if the *Faiona* is not here when she arrives we shall take her. The experience that we have had [shows] that we should have only our own folly to blame if we staked anything whatever on Grenfells carrying out any plan that he [had] made if at the moment, it did not happen to suit him. He does not take his life that way. He is in the midst of other plans now and would not let our convenience stand in his way for a moment.

This will bring us to Boston on the 9th of Sept. if we go by Battle and on the 4th, Monday morning early, the day that B. and the children leave Pasque, if we go by St. Johns, which on that count I am much inclined to do. I hate to go without seeing Grenfell. But I cannot let the courtesy cost me so dear. And there is no doubt whatever.... I do not mean that he wd. do it deliberately. But this is the way he sees everything and treats everybody. Everybody agrees, even those who love his work and honor him have learned to guide themselves by this trait.

And the Captain says with the simplest candor that he advises us against staking anything whatever on getting to Battle by the *Faiona*. It is fortunate that we have the *Lake* to get us out. And we must not let her pass us. When I asked in some solicitude before G. left what we could rely on he showed definite annoyance as if our presence turned out a hampering thing – as affairs have fallen out, and K. says he showed him the same mind clearly. The Captain says he said so in so many words to him.

I am sorry to go without asking Mays question about Dr. Runyon. But I shall leave a note asking it. Yet I could not advise a busy and responsible man ever to council [*sic*] himself to a cruise with G. without his knowing, at least, beforehand, how he might have to protect himself against emergencies.

Taking a walk with K. this afternoon we came by the pool where he bathed two weeks ago and there on the shore of it was a pile of man's clothing just as if a man had skinned out of them. We searched the neighborhood and did everything but drag the pool, but cd. find nothing. Then we walked back to the hospital and told Mumford who was all excitement at once for he said that a Newfoundland fisherman had disappeared here, three weeks ago, gone off to walk and nothing had been seen or heard of him since.

He walked back with us and looked at the clothing and searched the pool. The queerest part of it was that there were no shoes and no stockings, no coat and no hat. And the clothes had not been wet by rain – and it rained only yesterday – and indeed I passed quite near that place while walking this morning, and cd. almost swear that the clothes were not there. So finally we concluded that this was somebodys washing from one of the huts or a schooner. But why up there almost at the very top of a hill three hundred feet high I have no idea. We were convinced when we found more clothes actually laid in another pool a hundred yards away and weighted down with stones. So all our tragedy petered out.

Only Mumford said ruefully that it was from the little stream that runs down from those pools that the hospital gets its water. The water supply of almost all Labrador is from rainpools just like that. There is hardly a spring in a thousand miles of this coast. Why we do not all have typhoid I do not know. And in fact a good many of them do.

When we were looking for a place for the foxes – to leave them here – we looked in the cellar under the church, and there was a coffin of a man, a fisherman from the French shore, who has been laid away in salt, and the coffin covered with pitch waiting till his schooner goes home.

The clocks at the Hospital are an hour and a half out by our watches, and we have had no corrected time since we saw the *Faiona*'s chronometer two weeks ago. But among the fisher people and in such places as the hospital they do not get a correction on their clocks once in six months. So you can imagine what a variety there is and what an absurdity it is to try to make or keep an engagement.

Preparations To Go
Wed.[89] Aug. 24th.

Have decided to go by the *Lake* probably to St. Johns. Packing, long climb, very cold raw day. Fog at night. Dined at Hospital. Such a muff Mumford is. And such a fine woman Miss Williams. Prayed with old Mrs. Calloway who is surely going to die.

Going South By The *Virginia Lake*
Indian Harbor, Lab. Friday, Aug.25th.

All day long blew a gale of wind, sheets of rain, very cold, occasional fog – Half doubted if the *Lake* would reach us. But at 6:00 p.m. I saw her coming round the end of Cutthroat Island. She called at Smokey Tickle where the Marconi Station is and then ran into Bakeapple Bight for the night. Sent off a boat for the Indian Harbor mail and they bade us come aboard, as she would sail at dawn. We bade adieu to the good people on the *Strathcona* and went aboard about 9:00 oclock. We were fortunate enough to get berths, for she is very full.

On her deck we learned all they knew of the *Faiona* and the *Scylla*. The two ships had not met at all. But only day before yesterday, Wed. the *Lake* met the *Faiona* at Nain. She had cruised to Nachvak direct and after that hither and yon for ten days seeking the *Scylla* everywhere, and at last had to give it up and run to Nain for coal – where there was less than five tons by the way. A more disgusted and disgruntled ships company you can hardly think. For they had never had the gov. aboard at all and had done hardly any of all the things they had planned.

---

[89] Thursday

When the *Virginia Lake* got to Hopedale there lay the *Scylla*, with the gov. aboard. Gov. and Commodore also fuming and fretting. Gov's plans for observations all defeated, for the *Scylla* cannot run in to shore, and Commodore cursing[90] because he had had the Gov. aboard and…spent ten days of it hunting or waiting for Grenfell.

Now that the *Lake* had brought them the news of the *Faiona*, they wd. lie at Hopedale until the *Faiona* came – they would have to give her coal out of their own bunkers. Then both were to start south at once. Grenfell said they were to run straight for Cartwright from Indian Harbor where we lay, but expecting us to get the news. I suppose from the *Lake* and run for Cartwright too – But, he sent no order to that effect – no order at all. And meantime the Gov's private secretary who had been all this time on the *Faiona*, on his side expressed the opinion that, as the Gov. had much on his mind a visit to Rigolet and the time was now so fatally short, he thought they wd. drop Grenfell at Indian for his own ship, and run to Rigolet.

And since the Canadian Government's observation party is at Rigolet, they might stay there for the observation and so not come to Cartwright at all, but run straight for St. Johns. So much fault has been found with Grenfell's choice of Cartwright for the Lick Observatory party, as too near the sea and too liable to fog, that I should not in the least be surprised if they did do this. Then where should we be: if we had allowed the *Virginia Lake* to go by us? We should have to beseech G. to take us to Battle in the *Strathcona*, wh. after all his disappointments, he wd. probably have refused to do. Or else we should have had to stay in Cartwright two whole weeks waiting for the next *Lake*.

As it is we are off for the south, at last, and not any longer dependent on G. I never was more glad to get safely out of a scrape in my life. The last two weeks have been spoiled in Indian, the very thing which has happened to all his plans. It must be indefinitely humiliating to him. It certainly is an utter fiasco, the whole of his summer plan. And I cannot but think that – instead of ingratiating himself with the govt. and making friends for the Mission he has made enemies instead. And laid himself open egregiously.

---

[90] There was an old fisherman in Indian Tickle who could have taught the Commodore how to curse. When he was upset he would swear by stringing together the names of all the fish he didn't like: "Reevin' jumpin' Holy Moses, mackrel, sculpin, dogfish."

We shall stay on the *Lake* to St. Johns, arriving probably Wed. take the Thursday train and the Friday *Bruce* and be in Boston first thing Monday morning, 4th of Sept.

When we came to say goodbye to the Captain and thanked him for all he had done for our comfort, he said he was sorry it could not have been more etc. And added that he thought we must have had a most uncomfortable and unhappy time. He then went on to say that when there was first talk of the gov's trip, Grenfell had said that he was going to take the gov. and his sec. on the *Strathcona*. Bartlett asked him how he could, where he was going to get room. G. replied that he would send K. and me home from Battle Harbor, saying that he had been forced to change his plans etc.

When the gov. got the *Faiona* from the Minister of Marine and made up the larger party, G. was at first left out of it and was furious. All this time he never sent K. or me any word at all…. And the day we arrived at Battle Harbor, Sunday, and came across to the *Strathcona* from the dock as she lay at anchor, Bartlett says he burst out in the gangway where everybody could hear him, saying he was sorry he had invited us. Had hoped we could not come and now that we had come, he did not propose to let our presence in any way interfere with the important plans he had with the gov.

Now, I do not believe that the whole episode represents the least ill will on his part toward K. or myself. But it does illustrate how the last scheme wh. swims within his ken appropriates his [full attention] while it dominates him. And how regardless he is of any previous obligations incurred, and of any persons involved, if these seem to get in the way.

But at least I must be allowed to say that it has not been a comfortable situation. But rather one out of wh. I should often have given a good deal to escape. I have never before been four weeks in a house or on a ship when my room was better than my company. I do not believe that it wd. have been so had not this new dream chased before his eyes. But everybody who comes down here at all may make up his mind as to what he may expect, if it suits G's whims. And it wd. have been so easy to write to us explaining the complications and asking us if we cd. not come some other year or something of that sort.

There is a pitiable object on board, a man of 51 yrs, from Conception Bay, one of those who came down on the *Lake* early in June when she was carrying so many fishermen that some of them never even got below decks. It was bitterly cold. There were 270 aboard. These men were wet to the skin for days. All three had pleurisy and pneumonia at the Battle Harbor Hospital, two died and this one has barely escaped with his life. He has lost literally everything this years cruise, had a bad cruise last year. Could get nothing but a short job of cutting barrel hoops in the forest last winter, when for a month he slept on boughs and in the snow.

He has seven children, oldest fifteen, and he says had hoped to die. But now he must live and does not know what he is going to do. Is full of gratitude to the Hospital and Mission without wh. he surely wd. have perished, and no one can fail to see what it all means, or to give G. the credit of its organization and its sustenance.

But yet it is pitiful to see how impossible it is for any living being to live and work with him. Or how sharply he speaks to the poor sick people themselves, if he happens to be in the whim, how little he is beloved, how many enemies he has and largely by putting his own worst foot foremost and showing the petty side and the foibles and degeneracies of a great venturer living too much in isolation and too much in sole command and responsibility.

BACK TO BATTLE HARBOUR
S.S. *Virginia Lake*, Off Belle Isle, Monday, Aug. 28th.

Saturday and yesterday were as beautiful days as one could well imagine. We got away from Indian Harbor at 2:50 a.m. called at numerous stations all day long. Some of them we had visited more of them not. Was especially interested in the preparations for the eclipse at Cartwright.

Saw Swarfields little boy – the one who was bitten by the dogs. Only by the barest chance had Kingman met Mrs. Swarfield in Indian and given her treatment. She had come up to meet him but Grenfell had told him she was not coming. Could not leave home on account of eclipse, guests etc. She will have to go to Boston later on.

If ever I gave thanks for anything it was that I did not have to risk spending two weeks in that forlorn place just at this time of this year. It would have been worse than Makkovik for mosquitoes and nothing under heaven to do.

There are on board Mr. Elihu Root, the Sec. of State, and his two sons. Mr. Root very simple and affable, the sons nice young fellows, one of them most unfortunately deaf. Mr. Root very much interested in Mission and gave Simpson just now a cheque for $100.00 at Battle for the Hospital work. Interested in all that Kingman and I had to say of it.

Also there is with him a Mr. Sanger of New York, a Harvard man interested in Cambridge affairs. Convoying them is a Mr. Reid, one of the Reid – Newfoundland Company. And I suppose the ship is on its best behavior. But I am bound to say that if the table – e.g. is thus at its best, its worst must be pretty bad. Also there is a charming woman a Miss Linton who at once introduced herself to me as having visited Mrs. Cooke in Cambridge. Knowing Dorothea, and have attended my St. Johns School lectures last spring.

She knows a great many people in St. Johns, officials etc. is just going there for a visit. Is deeply sympathetic with Grenfell in his present bad luck and when she comes to Camb. in Oct. has promised to tell us what she hears. She admitted that Elihu, the governors sec. who had been on the *Faiona,* gave a most wrathful and disagreeable account of the whole thing.

Also there is a very nice girl, a Miss Hathaway, Assistant Prof. in Wellesley, who knows Miss Kendrick. She and three friends got off just now at Battle to wait until Sat. for the *Home.* They have enjoyed the trip immensely. We were able to arrange all things for them satisfactorily at Battle, tho. Simpson cd. not take them at the Hospital.

Sunday aft. a Mr. Carney, a Ch. of England Clergyman of about 70, a Cambridge man, Vicar of St. Marys Paddington, held service on deck as he had done the week before. A learned man and widely travelled very genial and progressive, sympathetic with America and knowing a great deal about it. Old-fashioned low ch. evangelical, deploring ritualism, worshiping Godit[91] etc. Took up a collection of 37.50 for the poor, sick man whom I mentioned just above – the Captains etc. in Indian had already collected and given him $43.00 – At this Service last week on the ship Mr. Carney had taken up a collection of 75.00 for Grenfells Mission. Carney knows all the Moravian leaders in England, too.

As it came night the fog came down and instead of reaching Battle as we sho. have done by 10:00 p.m. and running all night as the Captain hoped, we ran all night, or at least crept and crawled, and did not reach Battle until 8:00 this morning. We went to bed with our clothes on, expecting to be called at any moment: for I wanted to get my letters and my furs. But we might as well have undressed and had a quiet night of it.

I was on deck early and was in time to see the Captain make the Harbor in the most wonderful manner – <u>entirely by echo</u>. The fog was so dense you cd. not see the ships length. The ship had been running on and off, logging it, and then allowing for current all night. Dodging icebergs and sounding all the time. Shortly after I came on deck he blew the whistle and the echo came to us from the port bow – by wh. I knew that we were heading north. I expected him to put about. But instead of that he kept right on. By which I knew that he thought he knew where he was.

He kept testing it with the whistle, running very slow until presently he got the echo from both sides at once. Instantly he rang half speed ahead, and we slid along, the sound of the breakers on each bow growing more and more distinct and finally the white line of them on the rocks below the fog, on both sides became visible. Then still forward very slowly a little farther until an iceberg appeared exactly ahead of us. Instantly he ordered the anchor down and then we knew why the echo the last time or two had been so confused and seemed to come from all sides at once.

---

[91] Possibly the reference here is to clergy wearing—or in this case, not wearing—clerical regalia in worship services.

There we lay. A trap skiff or two passed us on their way out and said we were in Battle Harbor all right. And when the fog lifted a little there were the familiar converging shores – and a harbor full of ships – but – between us and them, lying exactly in the middle of the tickle and blocking the channel for so large a ship as ours – a large iceberg aground wh. had come in three days ago. It was the most wonderful feat of the kind I have ever seen. For we had not had a bearing of any sort since dark.

Went ashore after breakfast, took a patient, met Simpson coming out with two more whom he was sending away. Said goodbye to Croucher who had been very kind to us. Got my precious mail, four letters, bringing me down to 17th Aug. only ten days ago, got my furs and paid Simpson. Arranged for the young ladies to stay at Mrs. Esther Elson's. Saw Webster.

Had only just begun to read my mail when the call came to go aboard. Had not yet come to B's message about otter skin. When I read it it was too late. But I will write back to Simpson from St. Johns and he will bring it to Boston in autumn. In light of all the furs I have seen in the north, I am very well satisfied with my purchases and prices.

Just now we are passing under Belle Isle. We have passed four or five of the largest icebergs we have seen at all. One certainly 250 feet high and acres in area with a vast and beautiful spire. When you think how far south we are and how late it is – 28 Aug. – it is wonderful even in this funnel where the Arctic current does notoriously bring them – so indescribably white and pure, so little rotten or rounded off as by melting or wash. As if they had started from the Greenland glaciers yesterday. The French shore of Newfoundland is on our beam, and the Labrador is sinking on the horizon. Farewell to it. But we have had much joy of it.

The poor little French woman of the vast tumor is dead – Kidney trouble, autopsy showed it had been long present. Too bad.

Have just had a most interesting talk with a Boston man, a Mr. Cabot, who has spent seven summers among the mountain Indians back from Davis Inlet, studying language, habits etc. Has been with his canoe across the divide to the Georges River and down to Ungava Bay.

Explains such words as, Massachusetts, Connecticut, Narragansett etc. Country around big hill – Blue Hill – Valley of Long River territory from Mount Hope. Tells of the terror of the Iroquois memory among them – the Crees – to this day. Bad name for Newfoundlanders too, extinction of Newfoundland Indians,[92] not more than a few hundred Crees, in that whole vast area.

DISCUSSIONS IN THE SMOKING ROOM
Tuesday, Aug. 29th.

Gale struck us about dark hard wind and very heavy sea. Ship very light and high in water and pitched and rolled accordingly. Ships company pretty well laid out. Everything got about stateroom and for that matter, about decks, too, and the racket was unceasing. Worst was that somebody had asked steward to turn on steam so that the cabin was hot enough to boil lobsters, no ventilation whatever and no relief from the bad air.

Toward morning I went on deck. It was a great sight. Waves seemed to come sliding right down on us and it was hard to tell the masses of foam from masses of ice. We got a little respite from the rolling by breakfast time, and the rest of the day has not gone so badly. I have enjoyed it very much indeed. If only the ship were not so foully dirty.

Listened to the Captain talk in the Smoking Room.[93] He bears Grenfell a grudge for a time when it seems to him that G. exacted a very great price for [towing] the *Virginia Lake* from Francis Harbor to Battle when she had broken her screw. 850 pounds – he asked 1250 pounds, when the captain says he had said he wd. do it for nothing but the price of coal.

---

92 Beothuck or Beothuk Indians inhabited Newfoundland when the Europeans first arrived.

93 The Smoking Room was the social centre of all these coastal vessels. People spent many hours there and the conversations included all and sundry, and some said a lot there besides their prayers! I have experienced this on several trips on the *Kyle*. Read Ted Russell's poem, "The Smokeroom on the *Kyle*."

There was a running conversation among the others also as to the Coop stores and their relation to the traders and to the problem of the debts of the fishermen for advances to begin a new season when the previous season has been bad. Any one can see that Grenfell does not cover the whole case and that he has been pretty summary, and the traders feel that he misrepresents them.

Cabot thought he had been often rash and unwise but asserted utmost confidence in his good intention and ridiculed utterly the idea of G's doing these things for gain. That seems to be the prevailing judgment among those whose judgment is worth having, that he is a man of highest motive but not wise nor always just. Impulsive and unreliable often making representations and holding out expectations etc. wh. he cannot possibly keep…and dealing in generalities and assumptions.

If the Sandwich Bay location does not turn out well for the Lick people, as is now freely prophesied: it will be too bad one more case of the same sort…

Talkative old man, a man you can possibly think of, said yesterday of the old English Clergyman that he – the Clergyman – talked to everybody he could get to listen to him. Mr. Root winked his eye and said Boyle talked to everybody whether he cd get them to listen to him or not. Mr. Root talked of Russian, Japanese affairs.[94]

The Captain ended his speech by saying "This is the Mission ship this summer and there is the man who is caring for the sick folk this year," pointing to the ship's doctor, Boyle, who does indeed seem to be a very decent fellow. We heard only good of him up and down the coast, and he claims to have treated between five and six hundred people thus far this season.

He certainly is a great contrast to what the ship's doctors have usually been in their treatment of the people of the shore, especially to one who, a few years back used to drink like a fish and gamble aboard, and often refused to go ashore at all to see people when it did not suit his mood – though this was

---

[94] At that time Russia and Japan were engaged in discussions of peace. "In 1904 Japan took on the formidable power of Russia in Manchuria, defeating its armies on land and sinking not one but two of its fleets. In the peace signed in 1905, Japan gained extensive rights in Manchuria" (Margaret MacMillan, *Paris 1919*, p. 311).

what the govt. paid him for, and who ended by falling down the companion way and breaking his neck. He was the original of Duncans portrait in *Dr. Luke*.[95] But on the whole they have been a pretty uniformly bad lot until this man. And it was, no doubt, the competition of the Mission and the publicity wh. the Mission gave to such misdoings wh. led to the improvement.

There is a story which Croucher, the agent, told at Battle, of a Dr. at Twillingate who had a contract with a family for medical service – that seems to be the way here. Three children had the diphtheria desperately. He said that they could not be saved but by anti-toxin. He claimed its injection was surgical practice and not included in his fee.

The father said, Well, all right, go ahead. I will pay you when I sell my fish.

The Dr. said, No, cash down, or not at all.

The man raced up and down among his friends and borrowed $4.00. That wd. do for two. The fee was $2.00.

Well, said the Dr. wh. will you save.

The man begged him to trust him even only for this once for 2.00 more. He refused. They could not borrow more. They refused to choose as between the children.

He took a boy and a girl, and let the third child die. As he had previously let two women die in confinement because they could not pay in advance. The town held an indignation meeting, threatened to run him out. But finally settled down with an official record of the facts and their publication in the papers. The man left for awhile but is back again at his practice.

Boyle has had a case of confinement aboard yesterday. A girl of nineteen, unmarried, who had been a cook for a schooner crew, and was being sent home, as was supposed, in time. He said, and the captain bore him out, that while there are plenty of sad cases of girls who go up as cooks and are [decently treated] there are plenty more who go up understanding and the

---

[95] Norman Duncan, *Doctor Luke of the Labrador.*

captains take them of purpose for themselves or the whole crew. It is a state of things for wh. the Nfld govt has no law and concerning which public sentiment is very loud. He agreed that it was an outrageous state of things, and a great [insult] to all the crews. Poor old Mrs. Mileux at Batteau had it much on her heart.

Got a lot of Indian information out of Cabot who proves very interesting. Also about Hubbard and Wallace whom he knew. Travellers Club, Boston, photographs, slides etc. I doubt if any man living knows so much about these Indians who are relatively in their original condition. French Fur Trading Company etc.

Kingman conceived the sudden notion of getting off at Twillingate and making the cruise of Notre Dame Bay with the *Clyde* and landing at Lewisporte, and going by the little spur track to Notre Dame Junction to get the same train with us early Friday a.m. – 4:00 a.m. – I do not know what struck him. Whether the fierce weather we have been having, or the discomforts of our stateroom – wh. are supreme – steam heat, nearness of pantry, unspeakable filth etc. But I preferred to keep to the ship. I think there is no doubt we shall make the train at St. J. I shd. like to see the coast and St. Johns. I can imagine nothing worse than one of these coast towns and lumber camps.

And I think K. wished to avoid being drawn into Boyle's case. He had been asked to go down to see the patient, and had found the conditions nothing less than horrible. It was just at the height of the storm. He is very sensitive to such things. And it was not evident why he shd assume Boyles responsibilities. At all events he is gone. And we have passed a quiet and beautiful night, ran until 11:00 p.m. and then resumed at 3:00 a.m. Just at breakfast time – Wed. 30th – came on the eclipse.

ECLIPSE

Wed. 30th

It was gloriously clear. I hope it was so at Cartwright, and at North West River. We smoked glasses and used our spy glasses etc. and had a great view of it. Eclipse was, we estimated, say 7/8 ths total. and all the conditions were interesting. Of course I am sorry not to have seen it total. But even a man so used to all conditions up here as Cabot did not dare to take the risk of staying. Schooners were asking 50.00 a man, or 500.00 a schooner, and then might be a week on the way.[96] Mr. Root had seen two total eclipses and talked most interestingly of the experience.

All day we have had a beautiful run. Cabot has taken me into his room. We have taken on a very sick priest at Kings Cove, good part of his parish came down to say goodbye.

Boyles story of the intolerance of the ministers of the different Denominations one of another, and of the relation of the secterianism to the school problem etc.

Forgot to note once at the rail of the *Strathcona* where two small boys were looking at an illustrated paper, one pointed to two horses in a picture and said Them is harses. Ah, get out, said the other, how do you know.

---

[96] By way of contrast, note the following news item. "Solar Eclipse tour heads to Nunavut. – There will be an opportunity to view a total solar eclipse this summer – if you don't mind travelling to Nunavut. That is the closest place for Canadians to witness the 1.5 minute eclipse on Aug. 1, which will follow a path from Northern Canada to Greenland, central Russia, Mongolia and China. The Adventure Canada tour company is offering a six-day tour, from July 27 to Aug. 2, to experience the eclipse. It begins in Ottawa and includes flights to Pond Inlet and Devon Island in the North. The cost is $10,495 double occupancy" (*The Chronicle Herald*, Saturday, Feb. 16, 2008. p. E4).

A BUSY DAY ON SHORE
St. Johns, Nfld, Aug. 31st.

Long talk with Cabot, who has seen mostly small traders who were radically opposed to Grenfell on his Coop stores. With Root about educational esp. as affected by sectarian conditions. Representatives usually small St. Johns lawyers – not necessarily resident in district – Illiteracy 90%, so Mr Root says. This absurd state probably very wide at this time. About Japan and Russia, as also for knowledge of Hay-Bond Treaty.[97] Esquimaux women chewing boots, also chewing gum, also intoxicating liquor of Esquimaux obtained by chewed biscuits injected into molasses and water.

Passed life boat bottom side up with spars lashed on keel as if men had tried to hold on by her after she capsized. Captain held up and then proceeded on his way. Long delay at Harbor Grace in middle of night.

Arrived at St. Johns, Nfld, abt 7:00 a.m. Marvellous entrance to harbor, esp. from north. Bade goodbye to Miss Linton. Called later in the day at her brother in laws house and [said goodbye]. Went to Crosbie Hotel, breakfast and dinner.[98]

Cabot saw Job – with Job Jr. – Young man very frank and enthusiastic in support of Grenfell, even on traders issue, deeming that G. had done no harm to bigger traders, but had galvanized into moral respectability and

---

[97] Sir Robert Bond became Prime Minister of Newfoundland on March 7, 1900, and remained until 1909. John Hay was U.S. Secretary of State. The reference here is to their attempts to establish a Trade Reciprocity Agreement between Newfoundland and the U.S., which did not materialize at this time. Some claimed that Grenfell's descriptions of poverty in Newfoundland and Labrador influenced Americans toward a lack of confidence in the Newfoundland economy and they then refused to set up trading agreements. However, it is likely that the proposed Treaty of 1890 and 1905 was not ratified because Canada strongly opposed it for economic reasons, and there was stiff protectionist opposition in New England (various sources).

[98] There is some repetition in Moore's account of his time in St. John's. This is most likely the result of his writing these notes at two different times. The journals are also filled with abbreviated notes of certain topics and conversations.

debt paying, communities which before never thought of paying a debt. He had bearded in his den[99] the Bp of Nfld, Jones, for his censure of G. for his preaching in Wesleyan Chs etc. Gave high testimony to G. in commercial ways and had no sympathy with any opposition to him. Good to meet and talk with him…

I have never seen anything more full of life than the entrance to St. Johns Harbor. Bessie here more than twenty years ago. Day a full holiday. Not a shop of any kind opened, huge excursions. Nfld character affected by hardship, illiteracy. No admixture. Reid and politics. Miss Linton left at 7:30 p.m.

Most beautiful coast and esp. entrance to St. Johns Harbor. So glad Bessie has been here. Saw *Pelican* in Drydock, much injured. Hunted up Peters for Kingman's stuff. Saw the Capt. Of the *Blake*. Called on Miss Linton. Saw Mrs. Reid's little boys.

Nfld coast so much more varied than Lab. So very beautiful and rich, e.g. Tilt Cove and again St. Johns. Cabot's stories of Indian morality as compared with Eskimaux esp. in matter of women. Intermarriage among Nfld. People with absolute degeneracy is result.

Landed at 8:00 a.m. Thursday. All day in Nfld. St. Johns. Kingman's parcels and my investigation at W.H. Peter's, and Harvey's and Job's. Meeting of Lady MacGregor's coachman. McKenzie's journey in boat from Battle to Rigolet. Message to Simpson about otter fur.

---

[99] This means to confront a feared or influential person, to openly oppose or defy.

A Train Ride To Port Aux Basques
Sept. 1st.

Rd – Nfld. train late but hope still to catch *Bruce*. Train did not get away until 8 p.m. Instead of 5. Rainy night. Cool and dustless this morning, September 1st.

I have never seen anything more beautiful [than Nfld.]. Would not have missed either the coast from Twillingate to St. Johns or St. Johns itself for anything. Situation of the latter most remarkable. But town itself has all the squalor and vulgarity, brutality of the worst English towns. Eng. Cathedral is just about finishing repairs since the fire in 1892 when town was pretty much burned out Roman Cath. Cathedral not burned at that time.

Government House much like the fine old one in Halifax. Two or three man of war in harbor waiting for the arrival of the *Prince Louis* of Battenburg on Monday with part of the squadron. Commodore and Governor are due in the *Scylla* this, Friday, morning. This was the engagement wh. made it necessary for the Gov. to get away from Cartwright at once.

Mr. Root and party have a private car on this train. Mr. And Mrs. Bolles are in this car. Kingman expects to come aboard at Notre Dame Junction. We should have been there at 6:05 this a.m. It is now 9. The dining car service is very good. Road a narrow-gauge and unconscionably rough, lightly constructed, hardly secure for such fast running. Country largely burned over. Fire weed everywhere by the thousand acres on the burned patches. Saw two caribou on the edge of a lake.

Kingman did not come aboard at Notre Dame Junction. He had met Norman Duncan at Exploits on his way up with the *Clyde* and got off to spend a few days with him. You can think how glad I am to have escaped that, beside the pleasure I have had in continuing on the way as I had planned it. The two young men who went ashore with him brought the message.

Cabot's story of the case of gangrene of the lungs on the *V. L.* a few years ago, and the care of the ladies to illustrate the Newfoundland character. Very hard on one another. Lord Strathcona's past, his wife and son – Donald Smith – Esquimaux women, Esquimaux way of making intoxicating drinks.

All day kept losing time. Rained in aft. pools very full, road soggy, and country utterly desolate. So much of it burnt over. Came out abt. 5:00 p.m. at Bay of Islands. Humber River etc. very beautiful. Safely passed place of recent accident, and seemed in the darkness and driving rain to be running as fast as the wretched roadbed would permit, and yet when we arrived in Port aux Basques it was 2:45 a.m. instead of 9:00 p.m. Went aboard the *Bruce*, had a bite to eat and went to bed. Mr. Root a good deal disgusted at the delay. Parted with Mr. Reid, dull stupid fellow who had followed them the whole way…

CONNECTIONS THROUGH HALIFAX

Of course, we had long since given up hope of getting 8:15 train to St. John. No other train goes through to St. John until Monday a.m. No chance to reach Boston this way until Tuesday a.m. So I concluded to make reclamation on my ticket and go to Halifax to catch the S.S. *Halifax* of the Plant Line, if possible at 11:00 p.m. and so be in Boston early Monday. Literally nothing runs anywhere in Canada on Sunday. We shall see if we can make it. But the chances are good.

END OF THE TRIP

Bright day. Wonderful view of Grand Narrows and the Bras d'or Lakes. Telegraphed Bessie. News of the Russian Japanese peace.

Left North Sydney at 1:15 p.m. Got S.S. *Halifax* at 11:00 p.m. in Halifax. Made up bed in big saloon. Ship very crowded, most uncomfortable and demoralized. Rainy Sunday.

Arrived Boston 7:00 Monday, parted with Cabot and Mr. Cameron. Got furs through all right. Glad to be at home again. Telegraphed B. Go to Orange tomorrow.

BIBLIOGRAPHY

BOOKS AND PAPERS

Borlase, Tim. *The Labrador Inuit* (Labrador Studies). Labrador East Integrated School Board, Revised Edition, 1993.

Borlase, Tim. *The Labrador Settlers, Métis and Kablunângajuit* (Labrador Studies). Labrador East Integrated School Board, 1994.

Collins, J. J. "The Story of Marconi in Newfoundland," *The Book of Newfoundland*. Vol. 2. Ed. Joseph R. Smallwood. St. John's: Newfoundland Book Publishers, Ltd., 1937.

Duncan, Norman. *Doctor Luke of the Labrador.* New York: Gosset & Dunlap Publishers, 1904.

Gordon, The Reverend Henry. *The Labrador Parson: Journal of The Reverend Henry Gordon, 1915-1925.* F. Burnham Gill, revising editor. St John's: The Provincial Archives of Newfoundland and Labrador, 1972.

Grenfell, Sir Wilfred Thomason. *A Labrador Doctor: The Autobiography. Introduction by Sir Henry Richards.* London: Hodder and Stoughton Limited, 1948. This edition is an 'amalgam' of two autobiographies of Wilfred Grenfell, *Forty Years for Labrador* and *A Labrador Doctor.*

Grenfell, Sir Wilfred. "Labrador's Fight for Economic Freedom," 1927. *The Book of Newfoundland*. Vol. 6. Ed. Joseph R. Smallwood. St. John's: Newfoundland Book Publishers, Ltd., 1975.

Grenfell, Sir W.T. "The International Grenfell Movement," *The Book of Newfoundland*. Vol. 1. Ed. Joseph R. Smallwood. St. John's: Newfoundland Book Publishers, Ltd., 1937.

Hanrahan, Maura. *The Alphabet Fleet: The Pride of the Newfoundland Coastal Service.* St. John's: Flanker Press Limited, 2007.

Laverty, Paula. *Silk Stocking Mats: Hooked Mats of the Grenfell Mission.* Montreal: McGill-Queen's University Press, 2005.

MacMillan, Margaret. *Paris 1919: Six Months that Changed the World.* New York: Random House Trade Paperbacks, 2003. (Originally published in Britain in 2001).

Meaney, J.T. "Communication in Newfoundland," *The Book of Newfoundland.* Vol. 1. Ed. Joseph R. Smallwood. St. John's: Newfoundland Book Publishers, Ltd., 1937.

Moody, William R. *The Life of Dwight L. Moody.* New York: Fleming B. Revell Company, 1900.

Moore, Edward Caldwell. "Letters and Journal from Labrador," 1905. (Photocopies). bMS 422/7 and bMS 638/6, Andover-Harvard Theological Library, Harvard Divinity School, Cambridge, Massachusetts.

Penny, Alfred R. "The Newfoundland Railway: Newfoundland Epic," *The Book of Newfoundland.* Vol. 3. Ed. Joseph R. Smallwood. St. John's: Newfoundland Book Publishers, Ltd., 1967.

Poole, Cyril F., ed. *Encyclopedia of Newfoundland and Labrador.* Vol. 3. St. John's: Harry Cuff Publications Limited, 1991.

Poole, Cyril F., ed. *Encyclopedia of Newfoundland and Labrador.* Vol. 4. St. John's: Harry Cuff Publications Limited, 1993.

Poole, Cyril F., ed. *Encyclopedia of Newfoundland and Labrador.* Vol. 5. St. John's: Harry Cuff Publications Limited, 1994.

Rompkey, Ronald, ed. *Labrador Odyssey: The Journal and Photographs of Eliot Curwen on the Second Voyage of Wilfred Grenfell, 1893.* Montreal: McGill-Queen's University Press, 1996.

Smallwood, Joseph R., ed. *Encyclopedia of Newfoundland and Labrador.* Vol. 1 & 2. St. John's: Newfoundland Book Publishers, Ltd. (1967). Third Printing, 1994.

Smallwood, J. R., ed. *The Book of Newfoundland.* Vol. 1 & 2. St. John's: Newfoundland Book Publishers, Ltd., 1937.

Smallwood, J. R., ed. *The Book of Newfoundland.* Vol. 3. St. John's: Newfoundland Book Publishers, Ltd., 1967.

Smallwood, J. R., ed. *The Book of Newfoundland.* Vol. 6. St. John's: Newfoundland Book Publishers, Ltd., 1975.

Wallace, Dillon. *Grenfell of Labrador: A Story of His Life for Boys.* Toronto: McClelland & Stewart Ltd., 1946.

Wallace, Dillon. *The Lure of the Labrador Wild.* New York: Fleming B. Revell Company, 1905.

Whiteley, George. *Northern Seas, Hardy Sailors.* New York & London: W. W. Norton & Company, 1982.

PERIODICAL ARTICLES

Among the Deep Sea Fishers, 1903 to 1981. A periodical of the Grenfell Mission activities.

Them Days: Stories of Early Labrador. A quarterly publication since 1975. (edited by Dr. Doris Saunders until spring 2003, currently (2009) by Aimee Chaulk).

Toilers of the Deep: A Monthly Record of Mission Work Amongst Them. London: Royal National Mission to Deep Sea Fishermen, 1885 F.

WEBSITES

Andover-Harvard Library: www.hds.harvard.edu/library

The Canadian Encyclopedia: www.thecanadianencyclopedia.com

Department of Tourism, Culture and Recreation (Newfoundland): www.tcr.gov.nl.ca

Explore Labrador: www.explorelabrador.nf.ca

The International Grenfell Association: www.iga.nf.net

Lick Observatory, Mount Hamilton: www.mthamilton.ucolick.org

National Geographic: www.nationalgeographic.com

Provincial Archives, Government of Newfoundland and Labrador: www.therooms.ca/archives/

Science/AAAS: www.sciencemag.org

The University of Alberta: www.ualberta.ca

NEWSPAPERS

"Solar Eclipse tour heads to Nunavut," *The Chronicle Herald*, Feb. 16, 2008. Halifax, Nova Scotia. p. E4.

The Chronicle Herald, spring 2008. Halifax, Nova Scotia. (For discussions of mining in Moose River, Middle Musquodoboit, NS).

CORRESPONDENCE AND/OR PHOTOGRAPHS RECEIVED FROM:

Andover-Harvard Theological Library, Harvard Divinity School, Cambridge, Massachusetts. Ms. Frances O'Donnell, Curator of Manuscripts and Archives.

Tim Borlase, Labrador East Integrated School Board.

Sandys Moore Bureau, a grandchild of Edward Caldwell Moore.

Schlesinger Library on the History of Women in America, Radcliffe Institute, Harvard University. Ellen M. Shea, Head of Public Services.

Them Days: Stories of Early Labrador. ed. Aimee Chaulk. Administrator, Josie Lethbridge, Happy Valley-Goose Bay.

INDEX

ACKNOWLEDGEMENTS

I want to thank Ms. Frances O'Donnell, Curator of Manuscripts and Archives at the Andover-Harvard Theological Library, for her assistance in procuring copies of originals of Edward Calwell Moore's letters and journal, some of them typed, which I appreciated, and in giving permission to publish from Andover-Harvard Theological Library, the permanent location of these materials. I very much appreciate her help and suggestions in tracking down family members of E.C.M. Ms. O'Donnell also assisted by identifying, copying, and scanning photographs for this publication. Thank you, also, to Renata Kalnins, Reference Librarian at Harvard, for her help.

Thank you to Ellen M. Shea, Head of Public Services, Schlesinger Library on the History of Women in America, Radcliffe Institute (formerly Radcliffe College) Harvard University. Ms. Shea, after considerable effort, was able to get in touch with a grandchild of E.C.M. and to forward correspondence, which resulted in permission to publish these materials. Her prompt and willing assistance did much to facilitate the whole process.

Thank you to Sandys Moore Bureau, a grandchild of E.C.M., for her permission to publish, granted in the following correspondence regarding her grandfather's writings: "I am delighted that you find his writings about his journey to Labrador in 1905 of enough interest to wish to publish them, and I therefore give you full permission to use this material, as well as any photographs that are pertinent to your work. My cousin, Stark Ward, the only other grandchild of E.C.M., and I would very much appreciate copies of the book when it is finally published."

Thank you to all previous writers whom I have quoted: their acknowledgements are identified in the text. Thank you to my sons Daniel, for help with the index, and Mark, for help with the computer, and to my wife Linda, for proof reading and helping with research. Finally, thank you to Breakwater Books Ltd. for all their efforts in reviewing and publishing this work, especially to Rebecca Rose, vice-president, and Annamarie Beckel, editor.

Kirby Walsh,
Dartmouth, Nova Scotia.
Fall 2008

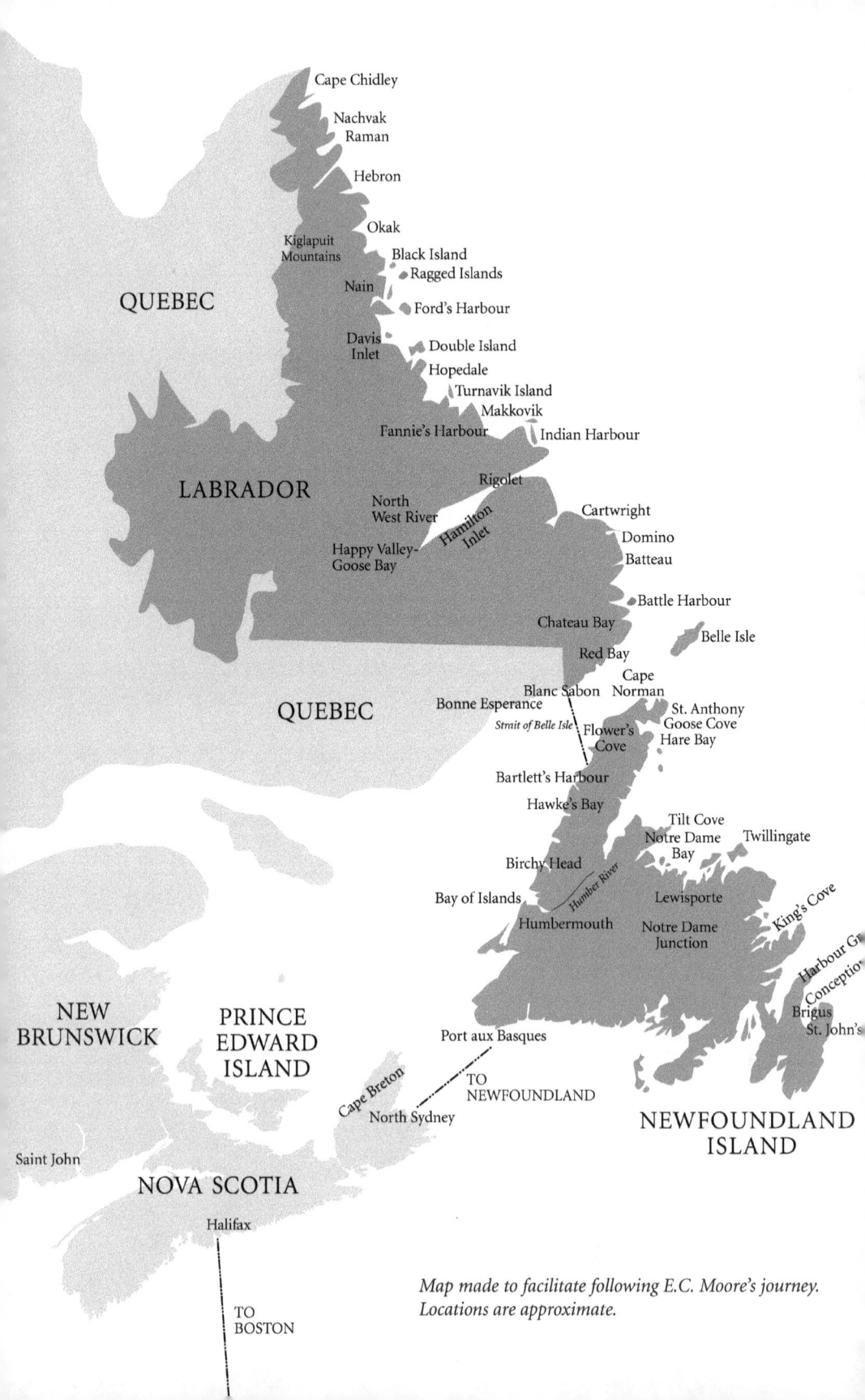

Cape Chidley

Nachvak
Raman

Hebron

Okak

Kiglapuit
Mountains

Black Island

Ragged Islands

QUEBEC

Nain

Ford's Harbour

Davis
Inlet

Double Island

Hopedale

Turnavik Island

Makkovik

LABRADOR

Fannie's Harbour

Indian Harbour

Rigolet

North
West River

Cartwright

Hamilton
Inlet

Domino

Happy Valley-
Goose Bay

Batteau

Battle Harbour

Chateau Bay

Belle Isle

Red Bay

Cape
Norman

Blanc Sabon

Bonne Esperance

St. Anthony
Goose Cove
Hare Bay

QUEBEC

Strait of Belle Isle

Flower's
Cove

Bartlett's Harbour

Hawke's Bay

Tilt Cove

Notre Dame
Bay

Twillingate

Birchy Head

Humber River

Lewisporte

King's Cove

Bay of Islands

Humbermouth

Notre Dame
Junction

Harbour Gr

NEW
BRUNSWICK

PRINCE
EDWARD
ISLAND

Port aux Basques

Conceptio

Brigus

St. John's

Cape Breton

TO
NEWFOUNDLAND

North Sydney

NEWFOUNDLAND
ISLAND

Saint John

NOVA SCOTIA

Halifax

*Map made to facilitate following E.C. Moore's journey.
Locations are approximate.*

TO
BOSTON

www.ingramcontent.com/pod-product-compliance
Lightning Source LLC
Chambersburg PA
CBHW072348090426
42741CB00012B/2973